Successful Posterior Composites

Quintessentials of Dental Practice – 32
Operative Dentistry – 6

Successful Posterior Composites

By

Christopher D Lynch

with contribution from Igor R Blum

Editor-in-Chief: Nairn H F Wilson
Editor Operative Dentistry: Paul A Brunton

Quintessence Publishing Co. Ltd.
London, Berlin, Chicago, Paris, Milan, Barcelona, Istanbul,
São Paulo, Tokyo, New Delhi, Moscow, Prague, Warsaw

British Library Cataloguing in Publication Data

Lynch, Christopher D.
  Successful posterior composites. – (Quintessentials of dental practice; v, 32)
  1. Dental resins 2. Fillings (Dentistry)
  I. Title II. Wilson, Nairn H. F.
  617.6'95

  ISBN-13: 9781850971207

ISBN-13: 978-1-85097-120-7

Foreword

The future of operative dentistry lies in prevention, risk assessment, minimally invasive techniques and the use of adhesively bonded, tooth-coloured restorative systems. An important aspect of the future of operative dentistry is the use of composite resins in the restoration of posterior teeth.

Composite resins for use in posterior teeth must never be thought of as a substitute for traditional materials; they are an alternative that offers a more modern, conservative approach to the restoration of damaged teeth, let alone being much more aesthetic than, in particular, dental amalgam. Furthermore, techniques for the use of composite resins suitable for the restoration of posterior teeth differ in important ways from the techniques for the successful use of composites in anterior teeth.

Successful Posterior Composites, one of the latest group of books to be published in the current highly acclaimed *Quintessentials of Dental Practice* series, provides students and practitioners of all levels of experience with a highly practical approach, based on best-available evidence, to the selection and application of composite resins in the restoration of posterior teeth.

Importantly, this book recognises that posterior composites are challenging, with consistent success requiring a good knowledge and understanding of the "where, when and how" of both the initial placement and post-treatment care of posterior composites in clinical service. All this and more is covered in this eminently readable, high-quality addition to the *Quintessentials* series.

Whatever your experience with posterior composites, this volume will expand and, it is hoped, reinforce elements of this important aspect of your clinical practice.

Mindful of the effective use of time required by busy practitioners and students, the author of this volume has gone to great lengths to produce a book that, in the spirit of the *Quintessentials* series, can be assimilated, with possible practice-changing effects, in a matter of a few hours – a great achievement in a subject area that is at the forefront of modern operative dentistry. For around the cost of one posterior composite, depending on size, type and complexity, this book is excellent value for money, let alone a great investment in keeping pace with the emerging future of operative dentistry.

Nairn Wilson
Editor-in-Chief

Preface

Of the many advances in the practice of dentistry, perhaps the most revolutionary has been the development of predictable adhesive techniques. One of these techniques is the placement of composite resin as an alternative to dental amalgam in load-bearing cavities in premolar and molar teeth. As a consequence, minimally interventional dental techniques for the management of caries in posterior teeth are a reality; for example, there is no longer a requirement to remove excessive amounts of intact tooth tissue to provide retention for "non-adhesive" materials such as dental amalgam.

Confusion has arisen regarding the most suitable techniques to use when restoring posterior teeth with composite resin. This has been a reflection, in part, of the ever-increasing range of commercial products available for placing posterior composites, a lack of consensus and educational guidance on the suitability of many materials and techniques, and a varied experience of success (and failure!) by dental practitioners in the use of composite resin in posterior load-bearing cavities. Failures associated with posterior composites are often attributed to a lack of understanding of the nature of composite resins, coupled with inappropriate use, handling and placement techniques.

The aim of this book is to give clear guidance to general practitioners on how to approach the restoration of posterior load-bearing cavities with composite resin. This guidance is based on current best available evidence. Above all, this book is intended as a guide for busy general dental practitioners, who may be able to browse a section during a break in a busy day in clinical practice. The structure of this book will allow the busy practitioner to read individual chapters as "stand-alone" sections.

Posterior composites are now an established feature of contemporary restorative dentistry, and are "here to stay". It is my sincere hope that all those reading this book will find it helpful and informative, and that they will come to enjoy placing successful posterior composites as much as I do.

Chris Lynch
Cardiff

For Catherine

Acknowledgements

I would like to say "thank you" to the following people:

Professor Nairn Wilson for his continual encouragement and expert guidance during the preparation of this book.

My first teacher of adhesive dentistry, Professor Robert McConnell, for introducing me to the concepts of adhesive dentistry and posterior composite restorations, and who has taught me never to be afraid to embrace new ideas.

Professor Robin O'Sullivan, who has been my mentor and friend for many years ... for teaching me that successful restorative and adhesive dentistry can only be truly understood in the context of oral biology, and in the structure and composition of the dental tissues with which we interact.

I am particularly indebted to Dr Igor Blum, Lecturer in Restorative Dentistry at the University of Bristol Dental School for writing Chapter 9; Dr Ali Kassir, Manchester University for Fig 2-3; Professor Robin O'Sullivan, Royal College of Surgeons – Medical University of Bahrain for Figs 2-8 and 5-1; Drs SB Jones and ME Barbour, University of Bristol Dental School for Fig 2-13; Dr Liam Jones for Fig 10-16. Sincere thanks to Mr Sam Evans and the staff of the Dental Illustration Unit at Cardiff University for their assistance in the production of many of the images in this textbook. Figures 4-7, 4-9, 4-10, 6-1, 9-2 and 9-3 are reproduced courtesy of Quintessence Publishing Co. Figure 10-6 is reproduced courtesy of *Dental Update*, and Figures 10-11b and 10-12 are reproduced courtesy of the *Journal of the Canadian Dental Association*. Thank you also to Ms Henriette Rintelen for producing the illustrations in this textbook, and Ms Mary O'Hara and the production staff at Quintessence UK for their expert support in producing the book.

Finally a big "thank you" to my friends – Dr Liam Jones, Professor Jeremy Rees, and Dr Alan Gilmour – for their suggestions, words of encouragement, and for reviewing this textbook prior to publication.

Contents

(all chapters by CD Lynch, unless otherwise stated)

Chapter 1
Posterior Composites: The State of Play
NHF Wilson and CD Lynch

Aim

New knowledge and understanding, and the commercial development of composite resin materials and associated bonding technologies, mean that the placement of composite resin in occlusal and all but the largest occlusoproximal cavities may, given appropriate technique, be considered predictable and effective. The aim of this chapter is to describe state-of-the-art approaches to the placement of posterior composites.

Outcome

After reading this chapter, the reader will understand how new knowledge and understanding and developments in the field of composite resin materials and bonding technologies have resulted in the predictable and effective placement of load-bearing composite restorations in posterior cavities.

Introduction

Attitudes to the placement of posterior composites have undergone significant changes in recent years. As recently as the late 1990s, guidance on the placement of composite resins in posterior teeth restricted the application to "small occlusal and occlusoproximal cavities in premolar teeth, and preferably in those with limited occlusal function". Educational surveys from that time demonstrated that most dental school graduates in Europe and North America had limited teaching in the placement of posterior composites, with many new dentists graduating with little or no clinical experience in their placement.

As a consequence of increased dental awareness in society, coupled with improvements in dietary and oral hygiene practices, many more patients, particularly younger patients, are now presenting with fewer and smaller lesions of caries than in the past (Figs 1-1 and 1-2). Such patients expect minimally interventive procedures, preferably using techniques that are described as "aesthetic" or "tooth coloured" (Fig 1-3). This, in association with commercial developments in composite resin materials and associated

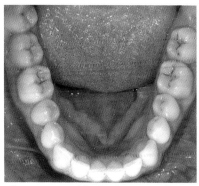

Fig 1-1 Mandibular dentition from a 30-year-old female, which is unrestored and caries free, albeit with some staining of occlusal fissures.

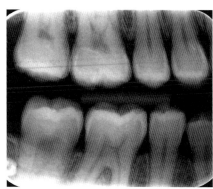

Fig 1-2 Bitewing radiograph from a healthy 35-year-old female demonstrating an absence of caries or restorations.

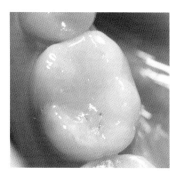

Fig 1-3 A recently placed composite restoration in the occlusal surface of a mandibular first molar.

bonding technologies and lingering concerns over the safety of dental amalgam, has driven an increase in the placement of posterior composite restorations in general dental practice. For example, a survey of United Kingdom general dental practitioners in 2001 revealed, far from limiting the placement of composite to small cavities in premolar teeth, that almost one-half of general dental practitioners placed composite resin restorations in load-bearing cavities in molar teeth (Figs 1-4 to 1-6).

With ever increasing patient expectations, coupled with improvements in the physical properties of composite resin materials and bonding technologies, it is highly likely that the placement of composite resins in posterior teeth will continue to increase in clinical practice.

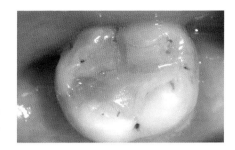

Fig 1-4 A posterior composite restoration that has been in clinical service for over eight years.

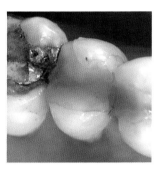

Fig 1-5 The composite restorations in the maxillary premolars have been in clinical service for over 10 years. While there is some evidence of marginal staining, the restorations are serviceable. This is in contrast to the deteriorating dental amalgam restoration in the maxillary first molar.

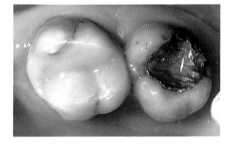

Fig 1-6 An extensive posterior composite restoration in a root-filled maxillary first molar. This restoration has been in service for more than six years.

Are posterior composites effective?

The answer as to whether posterior composites are effective is a resounding "yes". While some studies, dating back to the 1990s, found that the longevity of posterior composites was not as favourable as that of dental amalgam restorations, these studies investigated the use of composite resins as a substitute rather than an alternative to the use of dental amalgam. More recent studies indicate that the survival of posterior composite restorations can match, or even exceed, that of restorations of dental amalgam if they are applied to the best possible advantage. Indeed, dental insurance claims data in North America indicate that the longevity of posterior composites placed in general practice has matched and even surpassed that of dental amalgams. This has also been seen in recent studies of posterior restorations placed in general dental practice in Europe. Furthermore, as our understanding of the science of composite resins and bonding technologies increases, and practitioners become all the more familiar with the techniques necessary to place good-quality resin composite restorations, the survival rates of posterior composites will improve further.

One of the keys to success when placing posterior composites is to recognise that they are an alternative to, rather than a substitute for, dental amalgam and, as such, require very different operative techniques to those appropriate for dental amalgam. Dental amalgam is the "old workhorse" of operative dentistry. It is considered to be a forgiving, relatively easy material to place. In contrast, composite resins require meticulous attention to moisture control, must be placed using an incremental placement technique and are dependent on an array of equipment and devices including light-curing units, sophisticated matrix systems and multicomponent finishing processes, let alone the effective use of an appropriate dental adhesive. Notwithstanding these complexities, and the associated additional costs, the use of composite resins offers distinct advantages in clinical service over dental amalgams for the restoration of teeth damaged by caries and other insults.

Why is Composite Resin Better than Dental Amalgam?

Some of the advantages of appropriately applied composite resins over dental amalgams include:
- a reduced need to remove sound tooth substance in preparation
- opportunity to retain the restoration in non-retentive preparations through adhesive bonding to the remaining tooth tissues
- an aesthetic tooth-coloured appearance (Fig 1-7)
- reinforcement of the remaining tooth structure
- increased fracture resistance of the restored tooth unit (Fig 1-8)
- opportunity to repair and refurbish restorations in clinical service, thereby reducing the need for the total replacement of failing restorations (Fig 1-9).

Countering these advantages, there is evidence that posterior composites may be more susceptible to secondary caries than dental amalgams in cariogenic environments. Additionally, as and when total restoration replacement is indicated, dental amalgam, unlike most posterior composites, may be readily distinguished from remaining tooth tissue, thus limiting the risk of inadvertent removal of sound tooth tissue. As will be discussed later in this book, there are ways and means to minimise the effects of these limitations.

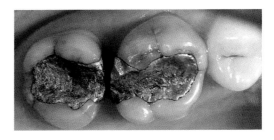

Fig 1-7 While these dental amalgam restorations are clinically acceptable, they lack the aesthetics increasingly expected by patients.

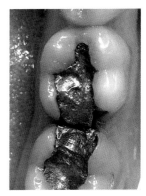

Fig 1-8 Fractured tooth tissue adjacent to an extensive dental amalgam restoration in a mandibular first molar.

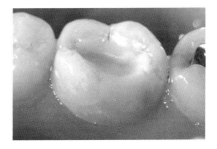

Fig 1-9 A repaired posterior composite restoration in a mandibular first molar; fracture of the distolingual cusp had occurred, and the area repaired with resin composite. A lighter shade of composite was selected to permit discrimination of underlying tooth tissue should further operative intervention be required.

The Way Forward

For many practitioners, there is a growing ethical problem. Is it in the patient's best interests to sacrifice sound tooth tissue to enable the effective application of dental amalgam, the tried and tested approach of 20th century operative dentistry, when it is possible to adopt minimally interventive preparation techniques through the use of a tooth-coloured alternative? It is suggested, as is now taught in many dental schools, that an adhesively bonded composite resin should be used to restore all but the largest initial lesion of caries, with particular techniques used if the preparation extends beyond the enamel cap, let alone subgingivally. Where dental amalgam has previously been used and the preparation may compromise the performance of a resin composite, as is often the case in the heavily restored dentitions of, for example, older patients, the reuse of dental amalgam may be the most efficient and effective restorative material. It should be remembered, however, that, once a preparation becomes complex and involves a number of surfaces of the tooth, an indirect cuspal coverage restoration will, in all probability, best enable the tooth to resist catastrophic failure under occlusal loading.

Given the above, it is apparent that a crossroads has been reached and passed in operative dentistry and the future will see continuing decline in the use of dental amalgam, albeit in some countries more quickly than others. Clinicians will need to move forward individually and collectively to work on continuing development in the application of resin composites and other tooth-coloured restorative systems. The goal is a style of operative dentistry that is less interventional and more aligned to the principle of the restoration of form, function and biomechanical performance of teeth than was possible with the approaches that dominated most of the 20th century.

Key Learning Points

- Placement of posterior composites in occlusal and occlusoproximal load-bearing cavities is now a successful and predictable form of operative treatment. Selecting composite resin for placement in posterior cavities rather than dental amalgam effectively increases the lifespan of the restored tooth.
- Composite resin is not "tooth-coloured dental amalgam"; it is an alternative to dental amalgam and as such it should not be handled or placed in the same way.
- Dentists should consider composite resin as the "material of choice" for the restoration of most initial posterior cavities, and should only consider placing dental amalgam in the continuing care of heavily restored dentitions, in particular in older patients.

Further Reading

Lynch CD, McConnell RJ, Wilson NHF. Trends in the placement of posterior composites in dental schools. J Dent Educ 2007;71:430–434.

Manhart J, Chen HY, Hamm G, Hickel R. Review of the clinical survival of direct and indirect restorations in posterior teeth in the permanent dentition. Oper Dent 2004;29:481–508.

Opdam NJM, Bronkhurst EM, Roeters JM, Loomans BAC. A retrospective clinical study on longevity of posterior composite and amalgam restorations. Dent Mater 2007;23:2–8.

Chapter 2
Let's Stick Together: How Do We "Bond" Composite Resin to Tooth?

Aim

Commercial and scientific developments have resulted in dental practitioners being presented with an ever-increasing array of composite resin materials and associated bonding technologies. The aim of this chapter is to review the means by which composite resins are bonded to tooth tissues.

Outcome

Having read this chapter, the reader will have:
- an appreciation of the range of composite resin materials available for restoring posterior load-bearing cavities
- an understanding of the significant properties and characteristics that should be considered when selecting an appropriate composite resin for restoring posterior load-bearing cavities
- an understanding of the processes of enamel and dentine bonding.

Ummm... Which Material Should I Use?

One of the keys to the successful use of composite resins is recognition of the limitations of the selected material. The challenge for the busy dental practitioner is to select the most appropriate material, bearing in mind that inappropriate material selection can lead to early failure. The purpose of the following section is to provide some helpful advice in overcoming this problem.

What is Composite Resin?

Composite resin is a combination of a resin and filler particles that are united together using a coupling agent.

Composite resins were traditionally classified according to the size of the filler particles they contained (Fig 2-1). This classification included terms such as:
- **macrofilled composites**, which include filler particles that vary in size from 1 to 15 μm and have a filler content in excess of 60% by volume

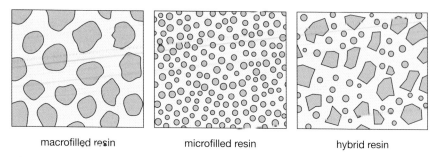

|macrofilled resin|microfilled resin|hybrid resin|

Fig 2-1 Differences in composition and filler sizes between macrofilled, microfilled and hybrid composite resins.

- **microfilled composites**, which include filler particles that vary in size from 0.1 to 1 μm, and have a filler content varying between 20 and 50% by volume
- **hybrid composites,** which include filler particles that contain a combination of microfiller and macrofiller particles up to 5 μm in size, and have a filler content varying between 50 and 70% by volume.

The properties of a composite vary according to the amount and size of the filler particles it contains:

- **Macrofilled composites** have a higher compressive strength and higher wear resistance than microfilled composites and hence are more suited to placement in areas where they will be exposed to occlusal loading. Given the size of the filler particles, it is not possible to polish macrofilled composites to as high a lustre as would be required in the anterior region of the mouth. They tend to be opaque in appearance and cannot achieve the translucent appearance that is required anteriorly.

- **Microfilled composites**, in contrast, contain very small filler particles and hence can be polished to a much higher lustre. They can mimic the appearance of natural tooth and are more suited than macrofilled composites to situations where aesthetics are critical. As microfilled composites have reduced filler loading when considered by volume, and hence greater resin content, they are not suitable for placement in load-bearing regions. They tend to have lower compressive strength and lower wear resistance than macrofilled resins.

- **Hybrid composites** attempt to combine the desirable features of both macrofilled and microfilled composites. While hybrid composites do not have the filler content of macrofilled resins, they have more favourable compressive strengths and wear resistance. As hybrid composites contain many fine particles, similar to microfilled composites, they are polishable to a high lustre and can, as a consequence, give good aesthetic results.

An important consideration when selecting a suitable composite material is the filler:resin ratio when reported by volume. It is important to realise that many manufacturers report this ratio by weight, which does not have the same implication for the material's performance. As the filler particles are heavier than the corresponding similarly sized amounts of resin, it is easier to "achieve" a higher filler:resin ratio when reporting by weight.

Newer Composite Materials
There are a number of newer types of composite.

- **Flowable composite resins** have a reduced filler:resin ratio (by volume). They are marketed on their ability to "flow" and hence are considered to be "easy to place" (Fig 2-2). Current evidence suggests that voids are relatively common between the restoration and underlying tooth structure when flowable composite resins are used (Fig 2-3). Such voids may, at least in part, be caused by the relatively high polymerisation contraction of flowable composites, linked to the large proportion of resin in the material. At one time, these materials were suggested as being suitable for placement at the base of proximal boxes in occlusoproximal cavities. Given the difficulties with voids in these materials, this is now considered inappropriate (Chapter 7). One possible use for flowable composite materials is to block out undercuts in the axial walls of crown preparations, but not in the region of preparation margins.

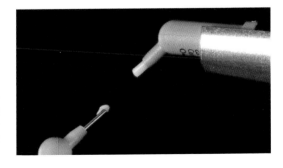

Fig 2-2 Differences in viscosity between flowable (left of image) and conventional/injectable composite resins (right of image).

11

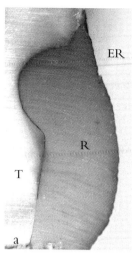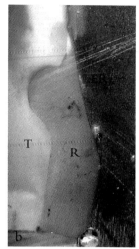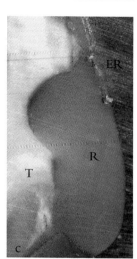

Fig 2-3 Stereomicroscopic view of the adaptation of composite materials in ultraconservative preparations in premolars: (a) flowable composite resins, (b) "injected" conventional composite resins and (c) condensed/packed conventional composite resins. These teeth were mounted in epoxy resin (ER), and sectioned in the mid mesiodistal plane. Leakage is indicated by the ingress of fuschin dye between the tooth (T) and restoration (R). This is most evident with the flowable resins (a) but least evident with conventional resins that were injected into the cavity (b). (Courtesy of Dr A Kassir, School of Dentistry, Manchester University.)

- **Nanohybrid composite resins** are showing a promising future. Nanohybrids, being hybrid composites, contain a mixture of particles including nanoparticles, which have a diameter of not greater than 10^{-9} metres (1 nm). This is in contrast to traditional micrometre-sized filler particles, which are over 1000 times larger in size. The incorporation of these nanoparticles increases the compressive strength of the polymerised material, as the nanoparticles impede fracture plane propagation within the completed restoration (Fig 2-4).

Making it Stick: Explaining Enamel and Dentine Bonding

The aim of this section is to describe the nature of enamel and dentine bonding. To improve understanding of these processes, it is helpful to review some recently introduced terms that describe available bonding systems:
- "**Fourth-generation**" bonding systems comprise separate etching, priming and bonding agents. These materials are often referred to as "three-

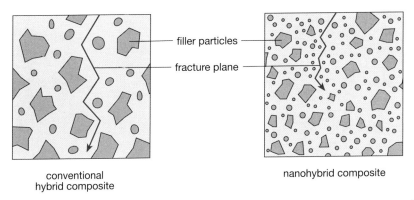

conventional
hybrid composite

nanohybrid composite

Fig 2-4 Illustration of how the composition of nanohybrid composites has improved resistance to fracture plane propagation in comparison with conventional hybrid composites.

bottle" or "three-step" systems (Fig 2-5). These systems are the "gold standard" against which other, newer, bonding technologies are compared. While successful enamel bonding was achieved using earlier generations of bonding systems, the fourth-generation systems were the first to achieve a predictable bond of appropriate strength to dentine.

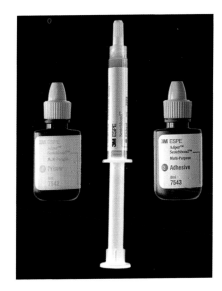

Fig 2-5 A "three-step"/fourth-generation bonding system. This comprises separate etching, priming and bonding agents.

13

- **"Fifth-generation"** bonding systems comprise a combined priming and bonding agent, together with a separate etchant (Fig 2-6). These materials are often referred to as "two-bottle" or "two-step" systems.

- **"Sixth-generation"** bonding systems contain a combined etchant and primer (a self-etching primer). In these systems, phosphoric acid has been replaced with a phosphate ester. Sixth-generation materials are available as "one-step" (Figs 2-7a,b) or "two step" systems, the former comprising a combined etchant, primer and bonding agent, the latter having a combined etchant and primer, with a separate bonding agent.

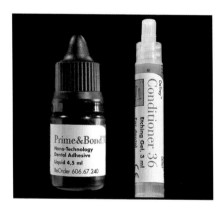

Fig 2-6 A "two-step"/fifth-generation bonding system. This comprises a combined priming and bonding agent, together with a separate etchant.

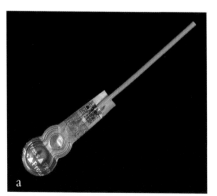 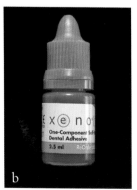

Fig 2-7a,b A "one-step"/sixth-generation bonding system. This comprises a combined etchant, primer and bonding agent.

Bonding to Enamel

Enamel bonding is a highly predictable operative technique. In 1955, Michael Buonocore described a seemingly increased "adhesion" of acrylic resins to enamel following acid etching of the enamel surface. To understand how enamel bonding works, it is important to consider the structure of human enamel.

Human enamel structure

Human enamel is a highly inorganic material, being composed mainly of hydroxyapatite crystals packed into enamel prisms (Fig 2-8). The prisms run continuously from the amelodentinal junction to close to the external enamel surface. The path taken by the prisms is not linear; they frequently decussate (bend) within the body of enamel (Fig 2-9). This decussation pattern results in the optical phenomenon of Hunter–Schreger bands, which can be seen in sectioned enamel (Fig 2-10). These are important when understanding how enamel bonding works.

Human enamel is mainly inorganic; it has no reparative abilities, is insensitive and does not contain any moisture. This makes it ideal for interacting with hydrophobic resins of the type included in resin composites.

How does enamel bonding work?

Enamel bonding works by resin tags interlocking in preferentially etched enamel prisms. The "adhesion" is effectively achieved using micromechanical retention. Enamel prisms are exposed during cavity preparation. Given the configuration of cavosurface margins, prisms are exposed at different

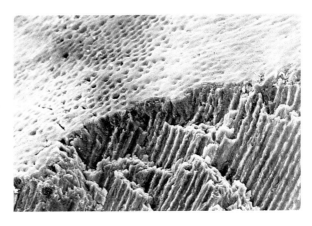

Fig 2-8 Scanning electron micrograph of enamel illustrating its prismatic structure. (Courtesy of Professor V R O'Sullivan, Royal College of Surgeons in Ireland – Medical University of Bahrain.)

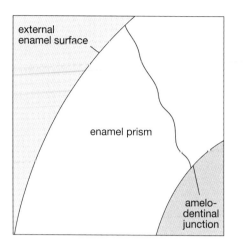

external
enamel surface

enamel prism

amelo-
dentinal
junction

Fig 2-9 Sinuous/decussating path taken by prisms as they move from the amelodentinal junction to the external enamel surface.

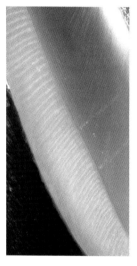

Fig 2-10 Hunter–Schreger band patterns in human enamel. This image is taken from the mid buccal surface of a maxillary canine. The alternating dark and light bands illustrate changes in prism direction. The frequency of changes in prism direction vary within the crown of the tooth.

angulations. This is most evident in the enamel found in the occlusal surfaces and coronal two-thirds of the axial surfaces of posterior teeth, where enamel decussation patterns (or Hunter–Schreger bands) are most frequent. When the prisms are etched, hydroxyapatite is preferentially dissolved from these prisms depending on their angulation. Prisms that enter the cut surface "head on" experience the greatest dissolution; prisms that run parallel to the cut surface are most "resistant" to etching. Most prisms are normally angled somewhere between the two extremes.

When using a fourth- or fifth-generation bonding system, enamel can be satisfactorily etched using phosphoric acid (usually 37%). This etchant is available in both liquid and gel forms (Fig 2-11). Liquid etchants flow more readily than gel etchants, which has both advantages and disadvantages. Using liquid etchants, it is easier to ensure that they have been applied to, and wet, the cavity surfaces and margins. From a safety viewpoint, however, gel etchants are preferable. Given the highly caustic nature of 37% phosphoric acid, the consequences of inadvertently dropping or splashing it into the patient's eyes are potentially serious. Intraorally, etchants can cause caustic burning of the gingivae. The use of a gel etchant, which is easier to control than a liquid, limits the risk of gingival burns.

Enamel may be etched for up to 40 seconds, though some studies have shown effective etching after as little as 15 seconds. Following this time, the etchant is washed away and the prepared surfaces air dried, giving the familiar "frosted" appearance (Fig 2-12). As bonding resins are hydrophobic and often viscous,

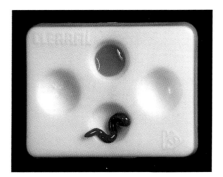

Fig 2-11 Phosphoric acid etchants are available in both liquid and gel forms.

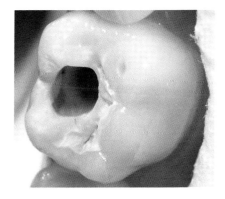

Fig 2-12 "Frosted" etched enamel surfaces.

it is necessary to apply a primer to the etched enamel first. The primer reduces the surface energy of the surface, encouraging the bonding resin to flow across and wet the etched prisms, forming resin tags Subsequently placed layers of composite resin, which should share the same chemistry as the bonding agent, form chemical linkages with the bonding layer.

Bonding to Dentine

Creation of a successful bond or "adhesion" to dentine was long considered an elusive, and possibly unattainable, goal. Early generations of bonding systems that successfully bonded to enamel failed to provide an adequate bond to dentine, resulting in leakage, post-operative sensitivity and recurrent caries if enamel bonding was incomplete or failed. The challenge of bonding to dentine was overcome with the fourth-generation bonding systems. Fifth- and sixth-generation bonding systems may be simpler and quicker to use than fourth-generation systems, but they may also be less predictable.

Human dentine structure

The structure of dentine, a wet, vital tissue, is dissimilar to that of enamel (Fig 2-13). Dentine consists of tens of thousands of dentinal tubules, which run from the pulp out into the body of the dentine and extend as far as the amelodentinal junction. These tubules contain fluid, odontoblast processes and sensitive nerve fibres (Fig 2-14).

In contrast to enamel, dentine, with its high-organic and low-inorganic content, has a reparative capacity; however, when repair occurs, this is at the expense of the pulp space.

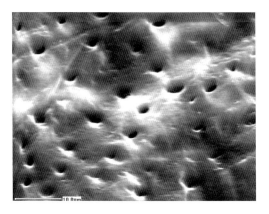

Fig 2-13 Scanning electron micrograph of dentine illustrating its tubular structure. (Courtesy of SB Jones and ME Barbour, University of Bristol, UK.)

18

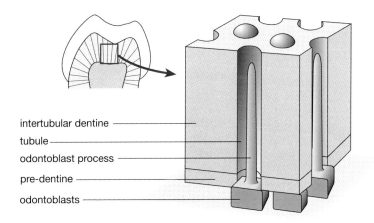

intertubular dentine
tubule
odontoblast process
pre-dentine
odontoblasts

Fig 2-14 Illustration of the structure of dentine.

How does dentine bonding work?
Following caries removal, the exposed dentine surface consists of a "smear layer", which covers the underlying dentine and occludes the dentinal tubules with smear plugs. Smear layer consists of:
• residual dentinal caries
• microorganisms
• collagen
• dentine chips.

As the smear layer is not a suitable substrate for bonding, it should be removed by acid etching. Current consensus is that etching dentine for a maximum of 15 seconds is sufficient. Following removal of the smear layer, a dense mat of collagen fibres remains on the dentine surface (Fig 2-15). For an adhesive bond to form, it is necessary for the bonding resin to infiltrate the collagen fibre. This is achieved with the aid of a primer, which "opens" the mat to allow infiltration of the collagenous network by the bonding agent. Resin tags also form in the exposed dentinal tubules, forming what is referred to as the hybrid layer (Fig 2-15). Dentine bonding, in a similar fashion to enamel bonding, is in reality a micromechanical retentive mechanism.

Considering currently available clinical evidence, predictable dentine bonding is now a reality in contemporary clinical practice. As this facilitates truly minimally interventive dentistry, the benefits for patients will become all the more apparent in years to come.

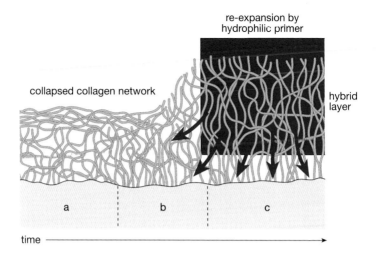

Fig 2-15 Formation of the hybrid layer. (a) The smear layer is removed, leaving a dense mat of collagen fibres on the dentine surface. (b) Application of a primer opens the mat to allow infiltration of the collagenous network by the bonding agent. (c) Resin tags also form in the exposed dentinal tubules, forming the hybrid layer.

Key Learning Points

- Always consider the properties of the composite resin selected for use; they need to be fit for purpose.
- Of the "newer" composite resin materials, nanohybrid composite resins have the most promising future.
- Enamel bonding is a highly predictable procedure.
- Dentine bonding has evolved to the extent that it should be in routine use.
- Fourth-generation bonding systems remain the "gold standard"; however fifth- and sixth-generation systems offer certain advantages.

Further Reading

Hikita K, van Meerbeek B, de Munck J, Ikeda T, van Landuyt K, Maida T, Lambrechts P, Peumans, M. Bonding effectiveness of adhesive luting agents to enamel and dentin. Dent Mater 2007;23:71–80.

Leinfelder KF. Dentin adhesives for the twenty-first century. Dent Clin North Am 2001;45:1–6.

Peumans M, Kanumilli P, de Munck J, van Landuyt K, Lambrechts P, van Meerbeek B. Clinical effectiveness of contemporary adhesives: a systematic review of current clinical trials. Dent Mater 2005;21:864–881.

Chapter 3
When Should We Place Posterior Composites?

Aim

This aim of this chapter is to describe the various indications for restoring posterior teeth with composite resin materials.

Outcome

Having read this chapter, the reader will be familiar with the various clinical factors that should be considered when selecting composite resin for the restoration of posterior cavities.

Introduction

A substantial amount of clinical time is expended by dental professionals restoring posterior teeth in the management of dental caries, deteriorating and failing restorations, tooth surface loss and the fracture of teeth. Each of these situations poses clinical challenges, not least of which is the selection of the most appropriate restorative material.

For some time, the dental profession has been aware that the management of dental caries should be by a "biological" rather than a "mechanical" approach. It is also widely understood that restorations do not cure caries. Controlling the caries process involves the cooperation of the patient in dietary management and effective oral hygiene practices. Furthermore, the decision to intervene operatively in the management of caries should not be taken lightly. The removal of tooth tissue in the placement of a restoration is irreversible, committing the patient to a lifetime of looking after a repaired tooth. Clearly, the decision to commit the patient to having a restored tooth, and all the possible sequelae that together form the "restorative (downward) spiral", should not be taken lightly (Fig 3-1).

Given the consequences of provision of a restoration, notably the inevitable weakening of the tooth through preparation, the operative intervention should be as minimally invasive as is compatible with an acceptable clinical outcome. The selection of the most appropriate restorative material should

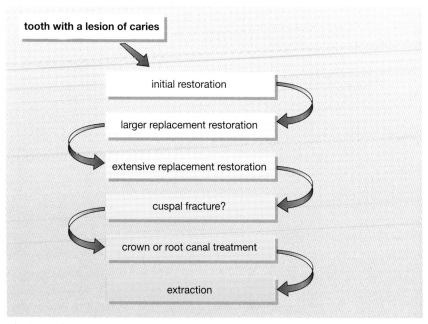

Fig 3-1 The restorative (downward) spiral.

be influenced by the potential to minimise the adverse effects of preparation, preserve pulp vitality and prevent further disease and damage to the tooth, let alone restore form, function and appearance.

Clinicians frequently ask "Which restorative material offers the greatest longevity?" While this is an important question, it is not as significant as asking "Which restorative material offers the most in terms of extending the life expectancy of the tooth?" The answer to this latter question must increasingly be a durable restorative system that facilitates minimal interventive dentistry based on a biological rather than a mechanistic approach, including the ability to bond to remaining tooth tissues and thereby offering advantages of marginal seal and biomechanical enhancement of the restored tooth unit.

Research evidence indicates that the longevity of posterior composite restorations has improved dramatically in recent years and in many situations has been found to be equal to, if not greater than, that of alternative materials. This, along with the continued development and refinement of composite resin materials and associated bonding technologies, let alone a greater understanding by the profession of the appropriate handling and use of resin-based materials, has led to predictable direct posterior composite restorations being a reality.

As discussed in Chapter 1, the selection of a composite resin to restore a posterior cavity confers significant advantages on the restored tooth unit. These advantages include:

- the ability of the material to adhere to the remaining tooth tissues, avoiding the need to create mechanical undercuts, and thereby limiting the size of the preparation and, in turn, the weakening effects of the removal of tooth tissues
- having the restoration adhesively bonded to the remaining tooth tissues, in particular the margins of the preparation, prevents the ingress of oral fluids and bacteria into the tooth–restoration interface
- being able to match the shade of the restoration to the remaining tooth tissues, thereby achieving an aesthetically pleasing clinical outcome.

Composite resins may, therefore, be considered to be the direct material of choice when adopting a modern approach to operative dentistry and, in particular, the management of caries. Alternative direct materials, including dental amalgam, should, in this view, only be placed in clinical situations where composite resin is contraindicated.

Where and When

While composite resins offer many advantages, there is a need to be aware of the limitations of resin-based systems in the restoration of teeth. Indirect restorations, up to and including full veneer crowns, still have a very large role to play in the restoration of teeth in everyday clinical practice. The indications and techniques for such restorations are dealt with in detail by Bartlett and Ricketts in their Quintessentials volume entitled *Indirect Restorations*. Where a direct restoration is indicated, as occurs in most situations, it is suggested that consideration should first be given to using a composite resin, and then to assessing the situation to determine if there are contraindications to preclude the use of such material. The contraindications may be considered under the headings of patient-based and tooth-based factors.

Patient-based Factors

There are few patient-based factors that contraindicate the selection of a composite resin for use in posterior teeth. These include:

- history of allergy or other adverse reaction to resin-based restorative materials
- the inability of the patient to cooperate with the placement of a posterior composite resin
- the refusal of the patient to give consent for the use of composite resin.

A history of allergy or other adverse reaction to resin-based materials must be taken most seriously. While allergy to resin-based materials in patients is rare, it can be dramatic, with possible life-threatening consequences. Patients who are or have previously been a member of the dental team may be most at risk of an adverse reaction to the use of a resin-based material, in particular if there is a history of repeated contact with uncured resins and associated local reactions.

In situations in which patient cooperation is limited and, as a consequence, moisture isolation may be problematical, it is to be remembered that the performance of dental amalgam, let alone other restorative materials, will also be compromised. In such situations, the use of a resin-modified glass–ionomer may be indicated in the provision of a transitional restoration to stabilise and maintain the tooth until such times as patient cooperation can be improved. Techniques to build and develop patient cooperation are outwith the scope of this book but are considered to involve more effective communication, educating the patient to understand better the need for their assistance in the delivery of effective dental care, and the phasing of treatment to establish and develop patient confidence. In the cooperative patient, techniques to facilitate moisture control may include patient familiarisation with a rubber dam, periodontal treatment to reduce false pocketing and the tendency of periodontal tissues to bleed, and crown lengthening.

Patient consent should always be obtained for any form of treatment. Although there may be good indication for the placement of a posterior composite, it is the right of the patient to decline such treatment. Alternative restorative materials and techniques should be discussed and agreed with each and every patient. A high risk of caries, let alone the presence of multiple active caries lesions, is not a contraindication limited to posterior composites or resin composites in general; it is an indication for caries control prior to planning any definitive restorations. Patients presenting with multiple, active lesions of caries should be entered into a stabilisation and maintenance programme, involving the removal of existing caries, placement of provisional restorations, dietary counselling and monitoring for the development of further caries. All these actions should significantly alter the caries risk. Once the patient's caries risk has been suitably reduced, then composite resin, or other restorative material as may be appropriate, may be selected for the definitive restoration of the diseased and damaged teeth.

Tooth-based Factors

There are no tooth-based factors that contraindicate the placement of a posterior composite resin restoration. There are, however, some situations that complicate, if not compromise, the use of resin composites in the restoration of posterior teeth. These include:

- development defects of enamel and dentine
- subgingival margins
- history of repeated failure of composite restorations
- discoloration of remaining tooth tissues.

The management of a tooth affected by localised or generalised dental defects, including amelogenesis and dentinogenesis imperfecta, centres around the capacity of the remaining tooth tissues to act as an effective substrate for an adhesively retained restoration (Fig 3-2).

Enamel and dentine of atypical composition and structure, including sclerotic and reparative dentine, must be assessed and possibly tested for its capacity to contribute to an adhesive bond. An assessment of bonding capacity may be undertaken by spot etching and bonding a small bead of composite on to the substrate and attempting to remove the material either with a hand instrument or with the use of an ultrasonic tip. Assuming the bonding capacity is found to be sufficient and an adhesively bonded restoration is placed, it is important to review the restoration at regular short intervals, at least initially.

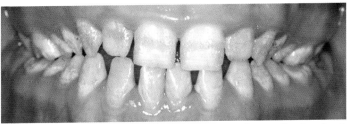

Fig 3-2 An example of amelogenesis imperfecta affecting both anterior and posterior teeth. These teeth need to be tested to assess if composite will bond effectively to them.

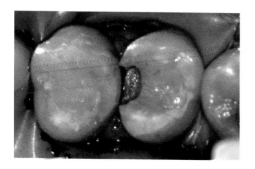

Fig 3-3 Subgingival margin on the mesial aspect of the maxillary second premolar. The problem of proper moisture control complicates placement of a composite restoration.

The presence of subgingival margins substantially complicates the successful placement of posterior composites (Fig 3-3). The skilful placement of rubber dam and a matrix may largely overcome the problem of subgingival margins, but moisture isolation may remain problematical. One of the possible options in such situations is the placement of an open-sandwich restoration, in which a resin-modified glass–ionomer material is used to restore the proximal box apical to the contact area prior to using a resin composite to restore the contact area, marginal ridges and occlusal portion of the restoration. Open-sandwich restorations are, however, at best long-term transitional restorations that facilitate other treatment such as periodontal therapy or possibly some form of crown lengthening to overcome the inherent difficulties of subgingival margins.

A history of repeated failure or repeated fracture may be a contraindication to the replacement of a posterior composite, but more often than not there is an undiagnosed clinical problem or a repeated error in the placement technique; for example, the restoration may be placed in too thin section to withstand occlusal loading. The successful management of restorations that suffer repeated failure can be difficult. To overcome the difficulty it is best to adopt a systematic approach to the assessment of the situation, starting with a critical review of the preparation followed by careful consideration of the occlusion. The possibility of two or more confounding factors must not be overlooked.

There are a number of situations in which posterior composites have been reported to have been successfully applied, these include:
- the restoration of carious lesions, including occlusal, proximal and multisurface defects and the replacement of missing cusps (Figs 3-4 to 3-6)

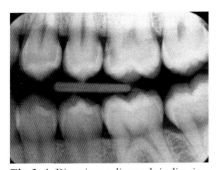

Fig 3-4 Bitewing radiograph indicating caries on the mesial aspect of the maxillary first molar that extends into dentine. Composite is indicated for the restoration of this lesion.

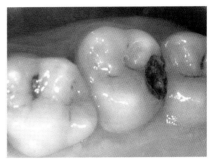

Fig 3-5 Dental amalgam restorations placed in maxillary molars where composite resin was indicated.

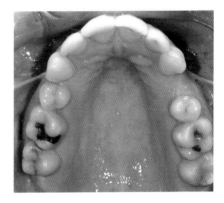

Fig 3-6 Another example of dental amalgam restorations placed in maxillary molars where composite resin was indicated.

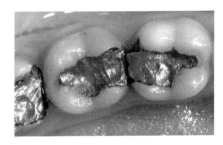

Fig 3-7 Secondary caries associated with the amalgam restoration in the mandibular first molar tooth.

• the replacement of failed restorations of alternative materials including failed restorations of dental amalgam (Fig 3-7)

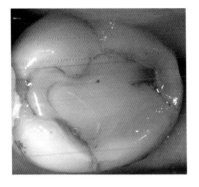

Fig 3-8 The ageing composite restoration on the occlusal surface of the mandibular first molar features some defects along the distal aspect of the occlusal surface. While the rest of the restoration is intact, it is possible to perform a localised repair of this region using composite resin.

- the repair and refurbishment of deteriorating or fractured restorations (Fig 3-8)
- the restoration of fractured tooth tissue adjacent to existing restorations, including the replacement of a lost cusp (Fig 3-9)
- the treatment of "cracked tooth syndrome" (Fig 3-10)

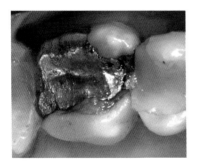

Fig 3-9 The dental amalgam restoration in the distobuccal region of the maxillary first molar has fractured. It is possible to restore this region using composite resin, thereby avoiding the need to remove the restoration in its entirety.

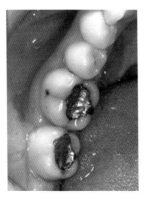

Fig 3-10 Examples of a mandibular first molar suffering from cracked tooth syndrome. The tooth has a large amalgam restoration, and stained enamel cracks are visible. The patient presented with a complaint of "pain on biting" and cracked tooth syndrome was demonstrated using bite tests.

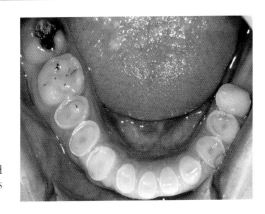

Fig 3-11 Worn anterior and posterior mandibular teeth. This patient had a history of bulimia.

- the build-up of endodontically treated teeth
- the restoration of teeth worn by attrition, erosion, or abrasion (Fig 3-11)
- the restoration of teeth that have suffered traumatic fractures
- the restoration of teeth to include retention features for removable partial dentures.

If composite resin is selected for placement in posterior situations, the challenge is to apply the material effectively in a way that restores form and function, preserves the vitality and integrity of the tooth and optimises the biomechanics of the restored tooth unit. To achieve these objectives, it is essential to have up-to-date understanding and knowledge of composite resins and the relevant operative techniques, together with an understanding of the biomechanics of restored tooth units. As the information on composite resins and operative techniques most appropriate for these materials continues to evolve rapidly, clinicians applying composites must keep abreast of innovations and developments.

Key Learning Points

- Given recent innovations and developments in composite resin materials and associated bonding technologies, the use and range of applications of posterior composites is now extensive.
- The use of dental amalgam or other alternative direct restorative material should be considered only when there is a valid contraindication to the use of an adhesively bonded posterior composite.

- The use of composite resin in the restoration of posterior teeth provides the best opportunity for the adoption of a minimally interventive approach.

Further Reading

Manhart J, Chen HY, Hamm G, Hickel R. Review of the clinical survival of direct and indirect restorations in posterior teeth in the permanent dentition. Oper Dent 2004;29:481–508.

Opdam NJM, Bronkhurst EM, Roeters JM, Loomans BAC. A retrospective clinical study on longevity of posterior composite and amalgam restorations. Dent Mater 2007;23:2–8.

Chapter 4

Getting Ready: Cavities for Posterior Composites

Aim

The aim of this chapter is to review contemporary guidance on preparing cavities in posterior teeth to facilitate the placement of composite resin restorations.

Outcome

At the end of this chapter the reader will:
- be aware of how patterns of dental disease, including dental caries, are continuously changing
- appreciate the various techniques presently available for diagnosing and treating dental caries, with an emphasis on modern, minimally interventive approaches
- be aware of the specific design features of cavities for posterior composites
- appreciate the need for adequate isolation prior to placing posterior composite restorations.

Introduction

The patterns of dental disease, including dental caries, are changing. Surveys of dental health in many western countries show an overall decrease in the levels of dental caries, while more notably, there is increased tooth retention. This is most marked in regions where water is fluoridated. Other factors include improved oral hygiene practices, more uptake of regular dental care, increased affluence in society and greater dental awareness amongst the population. As a consequence, patterns of dental caries are changing. Two general patterns are emerging:
- the occurrence of relatively small occlusal and proximal lesions of caries in patients with dentitions that are otherwise relatively disease free; the lesions are usually in younger patients and are caused by inadequate oral hygiene practices, inappropriate diet or a combination of these factors

- recurrence or new disease associated with existing restorations, typically in heavily restored dentitions; this presentation of caries is anticipated to become more common in years to come as more ageing patients retain more teeth, many of which are restored with traditional materials, notably dental amalgam.

Clearly, the emerging presentations of caries are very different to disease patterns of the past, when many patients presented with multiple and often grossly carious teeth. The changing clinical scenarios place different demands on dental practitioners when diagnosing and treating caries, let alone other damage to teeth.

In identifying new patterns of caries in younger and older patients, it is acknowledged that there will continue to be patients, from socially deprived groups in particular, who will present with more traditional presentations of active, uncontrolled caries. The management of such patients, which should be driven by preventive factors, deserves special consideration outwith the scope of the present book. The restoration of teeth in such patients may well involve the use of resin composites, but not until such times as acute treatment needs have been met and the dental caries has been brought under control. This is the approach to be adopted in such patients, irrespective of plans for the long-term restoration of the teeth.

A Review of the Carious Process

The purpose of this textbook does not include a detailed consideration of the aetiology and development of dental caries. No consideration of the design of cavities for restorations could, however, be complete without including a brief review of the process of formation and development of lesions of dental caries. This process is especially significant for posterior composite restorations, as cavities for such restorations are increasingly limited to the extent of the caries lesion.

Dental caries has a multifactorial aetiology, its initiation and progression depending upon an interaction between four independent factors (Fig 4-1):
- **bacterial plaque**, containing most notably streptococci of the *mutans* group
- **fermentable carbohydrates**, which are metabolised by bacteria to produce acid
- a **susceptible tooth surface** that is difficult to clean because of its shape or location

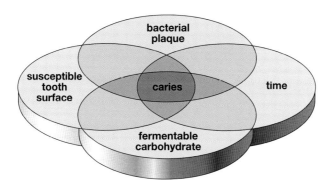

Fig 4-1 Schematic illustration of the aetiology of caries.

- **time**, the longer the tooth surface is exposed to the acid, the more likely it is that caries will be initiated.

Intake of food substances such as sugar introduces fermentable carbohydrates to the oral environment. Bacterial plaque metabolise these sugars to produce acid, which in a matter of minutes can cause the local pH to fall quite dramatically. The production of saliva, which contains alkaline buffers, returns the oral pH to "normal", but during the 30–60 minutes it takes to do so, susceptible tooth surfaces undergo demineralisation, which heralds the initiation or progression of dental caries (Fig 4-2). It will be appreciated that the frequency of intake of fermentable carbohydrates can promote the creation of an environment favourable to the initiation of dental caries to a greater extent than the amounts of carbohydrate ingested.

The absence or removal of one of the four key factors will both prevent the initiation of dental caries and modify the development of existing lesions. Examples include:
- excluding or reducing the frequency of intake of fermentable carbohydrates, such as sugars, from the diet
- mechanical removal of bacterial plaque, usually by tooth brushing and flossing
- the introduction of fluoride to the oral environment, in the form of rinses, additions to foodstuffs or as fluoridation of water sources.

The advantages conferred by fluoride include:
- the "strengthening" of surface enamel by replacing hydroxyapatite with fluorapatite, which is more resistant to acidic dissolution

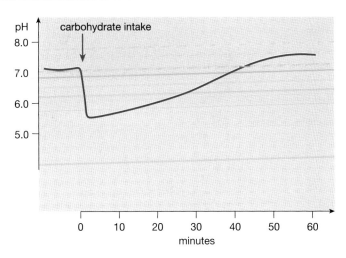

Fig 4-2 The effect of carbohydrate intake on the oral pH (the Stephan curve).

- the ability to damage and destroy many cariogenic bacteria
- the ability to reverse the fall in the oral pH quickly following the ingestion of fermentable carbohydrates, though this is only possible if fluoride is introduced to the oral cavity at the same time or shortly after the ingestion of these sugars.

The rate and nature of development of caries is influenced by diet, cleaning and the availability of fluoride. In modern society, caries, where present, progresses relatively slowly and, as a consequence, when first diagnosed is not well advanced, unless of course, previous diagnosis has been ineffective.

Techniques for Diagnosing Dental Caries: Are We Really Sure It's There?

When planning to perform any form of treatment, it is essential to diagnose the presence of a disease accurately and to assess its level of activity and likelihood of progression. When seeking a diagnosis of dental caries, it is essential initially to obtain and record an accurate history from the patient. This will give clues as to the possible presence, nature and activity of any disease. Important information to be recorded includes:

- the nature, duration, and frequency of any dental pain, or discomfort
- the dietary habits of the patient, including the frequency and intake of fermentable carbohydrates

- the frequency of dental attendance and the dental history
- the oral hygiene practices of the patient, including the frequency of toothbrushing, the use of dental floss and other oral hygiene aids
- the presence of any medical conditions that may modify the disease susceptibility and process.

The development of dental caries can be influenced by certain medications, for example diminishing salivary flow; by certain disorders, for example neuromuscular disorders or conditions such as rheumatoid arthritis may limit the patient's ability to maintain adequate oral hygiene; and by a multiplicitiy of conditions that may influence diet, notably the frequency of the intake of fermentable carbohydrates.

Following collection of all relevant information, it is necessary to examine the dentition for the presence and activity of dental caries. Methods for achieving this include:
- visual examination
- transillumination
- radiographic examination
- caries detection dyes
- electrical conductance methods
- fluorescence methods.

Visual Examination

Visual examination of suspect teeth should be the first investigation for dental caries. In keeping with current best-available evidence, teeth should be cleaned, dried and inspected under a bright light, preferably using magnification (Figs 4-3 and 4-4).

Particular attention should be paid to the occlusal and proximal surfaces of the teeth (Figs 4-5 and 4-6). Given typical oral hygiene and dietary practices in modern society, occlusal caries may be very difficult to detect visually, as the only obvious clinical signs are the presence of shadowing and discrete decalcified areas on or near the occlusal fissures (Fig 4-6). The use of dental explorers to investigate any suspected fissure or defect in enamel is contraindicated, as this can damage the enamel, allowing initiation or progression of early dental caries.

If caries is suspected to be present, further diagnostic tests must be applied. No one diagnostic technique is sufficiently sensitive, let alone specific enough, to be relied on as the sole means of diagnosis, except when the lesion is extensive, particularly following cavitation.

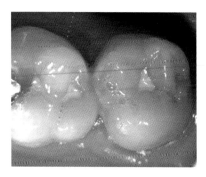

Fig 4-3 It is difficult to examine the occlusal surface without first drying the area.

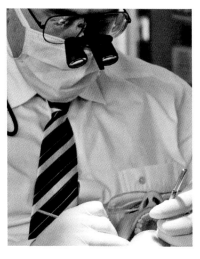

Fig 4-4 Magnification is a useful tool when examining suspect areas.

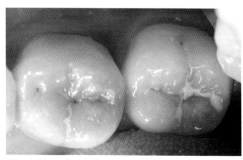

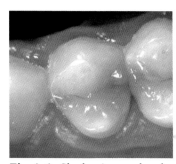

Fig 4-5 Is the defect on the occlusal surface of the mandibular first molar carious? Does the shadowing under the occlusal surface of this mandibular first molar indicate the need for operative intervention?

Fig 4-6 Shadowing under the distal marginal ridge area of a maxillary left first premolar. Does this indicate the presence of caries?

Transillumination

Transillumination of suspected teeth is a useful technique in the diagnosis of dental caries. This involves the use of pencil beams of visible light to demonstrate the presence of lesions of caries, and other defects such as enamel cracks. Special transilluminating and fibre-optic lights have been developed for this purpose. Visible light-curing units should not be used for this purpose as this entails looking at light that could cause retinal damage. If used appropriately, and according to best practice, transillumination can be a very helpful adjunct to the effective diagnosis of caries (Fig 4-7).

Radiographic Examination

Radiographic examination of suspect teeth is indicated, particularly if transillumination examination has indicated the possible presence of lesions. The most appropriate form of radiographic examination for the presence of dental caries in posterior teeth is the bitewing view. Information collected in this way should, however, be considered together with information collected during the patient's history, the visual examination and trans-illumination before arriving at a diagnosis.

Bitewing radiographs are more sensitive at diagnosing lesions of caries in proximal rather than occlusal surfaces, given the complex morphology of occlusal surfaces (Fig 4-8). Bitewing radiographs should be taken using an appropriate beam-directing device. This limits the superimposition of proximal surfaces.

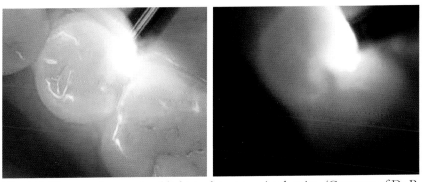

Fig 4-7 The use of transmitted light to detect proximal caries. (Courtesy of Dr R Trushkowsky; from NHF Wilson, *Minimally Invasive Dentistry*. London: Quintessence, 2007.)

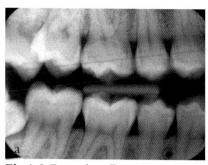 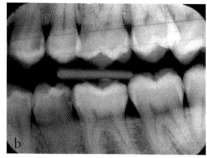

Fig 4-8 Examples of bitewing radiographs taken from a 32-year-old female patient. Several proximal lesions of caries are visible. The image in (b) shows distal caries in the maxillary left first premolar; this is the same tooth as shown in Fig 4-6.

Caries Detection Dyes

Caries detection dyes are of limited use when attempting to detect and diagnose caries. While the use of dyes has been reported to be of some use in the diagnosis of residual dentinal caries in cavity preparations, the use of dyes for detecting enamel caries is limited. Dyes used to detect enamel caries often cause unacceptable irreversible staining, and they may lead to false-positive results. Such dyes are of little use in the initial clinical examination of patients.

Electrical Conductance Methods

Electrical conductance methods utilise a small electrical current passed through a suspected tooth. The presence of dental caries alters the electrical resistance of the tooth to an extent that can be recorded. While this technique is good for detecting early lesions, it can be "over-sensitive", sometimes incorrectly identifying sound teeth as being diseased.

Fluorescence Methods

The use of fluorescence methods to detect caries has generated renewed interest recently. The technique is based on the differential absorption of light by carious and healthy dental hard tissues. Absorption of light moves electrons in a lower energy level to a higher energy level; when these fall back to their original level, energy is emitted in the form of light fluorescence. A difference in fluorescence radiance between carious and healthy tooth structure can be measured and used to detect and quantify caries.

Two fluorescence techniques have been described to date: quantitative light-induced fluorescence (QLF) and DIAGNOdent (KaVo, Biberach, Germany). While QLF can successfully detect smooth surface lesions of caries, its

40

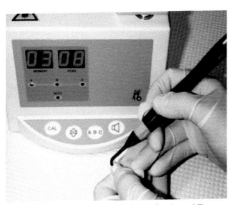

Fig 4-9 The DIAGNOdent device. (Courtesy of Xie-Qi Shi et al; from NHF Wilson, *Minimally Invasive Dentistry*. London: Quintessence, 2007.)

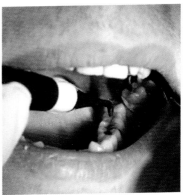

Fig 4-10 Clinical use of DIAGNOdent. (Courtesy of Xie-Qi Shi et al; from NHF Wilson, *Minimally Invasive Dentistry*. London: Quintessence, 2007.)

application seems to be limited to a lesion depth of approximately 500 μm. Its use in the detection of occlusal caries remains to be fully investigated. DIAGNOdent, however, offers a promising means of predictable, non-invasive, caries detection. DIAGNOdent is a laser-based instrument that measures differences in the fluorescence of suspect dental tissues irradiated with red light. It can be used to detect caries in both smooth and occlusal surfaces. Recent investigations have indicated that DIAGNOdent could be as reliable as bitewing radiography in diagnosing occlusal caries. The DIAGNOdent instrument comprises a descending fibre that transmits laser light to the suspect surface and an ascending fibre that transmits fluorescence to a photodiode detector. The signal is presented as an integer on the display of the measuring device. This device shows promise as a truly minimal intervention to diagnose caries; readers, if not persuaded to invest in this technology, are encouraged to follow the future development of DIAGNOdent in coming years (Figs 4-9 and 4-10).

New Ways to Approach an Old Problem: Caries Management Strategies for Today

Risk Assessment

With changing therapeutic paradigms, it is recognised that it is not always necessary to restore every tooth affected by caries. It is essential to recognise cavity preparation as an irreversible process that substantially weakens teeth

41

and, once initiated, commits the tooth to a lifetime of maintenance and operative treatment. While it was once recognised that the presence of caries at, or anywhere beyond, the amelodentinal junction was an absolute indication for operative treatment, this philosophy has undergone further refinement. It is now understood that individual lesions should be assessed for likely risk of progression. This is best understood by comparing the following clinical examples:

- a 15-year-old patient, with a large mesio-occlusal lesion of caries in the mandibular left second premolar, with the caries well into dentine; the patient has eight existing restorations, is an irregular dental attender and has a high plaque score
- a 45-year-old patient who has a small lesion of caries on the palatal surface in the maxillary right first molar, with the caries extending just beyond the amelodentinal junction; the patient has four restored teeth, attends a dentist on an annual basis and has good plaque control.

Clearly the first patient is at a greater risk of caries progression and is in greater need of operative intervention. The lesion in the second patient may best be managed by preventive measures and monitoring.

Factors to consider when making a caries risk assessment include:
- the patient's diet, including the frequency and consumption of fermentable carbohydrates
- the adequacy of the patient's oral hygiene practices, and the use of fluoride
- the volume and quality of saliva
- the patient's socioeconomic status
- previous evidence of dental caries, as evidenced by the numbers of decayed, restored and missing teeth
- current disease activity, as evidenced by the numbers of active lesions of caries present
- attendance habits for dental check-ups
- other confounding factors.

Mechanical Caries Removal

The process of removing dentinal caries mechanically is a long-established technique in operative dentistry (Figs 4-11 and 4-12). It is still the quickest means of removing caries but it can often result in the excessive removal of healthy dentine and, when managing proximal lesions, invariably results in iatrogenic damage to adjacent teeth. When mechanical caries removal is being performed, it is recommended that caries on the walls of the cavity is removed

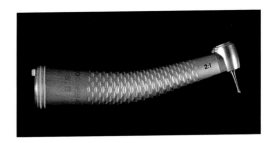

Fig 4-11 Slow handpiece with round stainless steel bur for mechanical caries removal.

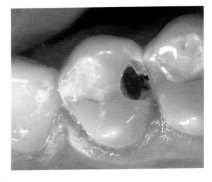

Fig 4-12 The image here is of the same tooth as shown in Figs 4-6 and 4-8b. Following removal of the surface enamel, the dentinal caries is exposed. Interestingly, this image shows a discoloured enamel region on the distal surface; this lesion corresponds to the radiolucent "break" in the enamel shown in the maxillary first premolar in Fig 4-8b.

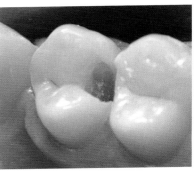

Fig 4-13 Caries should be removed from the walls of the cavity before being removed from the floor. This image shows unsupported enamel on the buccal wall. There is no requirement to remove this for composite restorations; however, if an amalgam restoration were being placed, this healthy tissue would be sacrificed.

before attempting to remove caries from the pulpal floor (Fig 4-13). When removing caries prior to the placement of a posterior composite, it is not always necessary to cut or excavate back to sound dentine. If the caries is very deep and further removal may involve the pulp, either directly or indirectly, then some softened, unstained dentine may be left in the base of the cavity. Removing caries by means of a diamond bur, which tends to shatter rather than cut through enamel, can lead to the formation of a thick smear layer and the generation of more heat than caused by a tungsten carbide fluted bur.

43

Chemomechanical Caries Removal

Chemomechanical caries removal techniques were developed as an alternative to traditional mechanical techniques. The chemomechanical methods are based on the principle of applying a special gel or liquid (e.g. Carisolv) that selectively softens carious dentine prior to its mechanical removal with specially designed hand instruments. Chemomechanical removal offers a number of distinct advantages over traditional mechanical techniques, including:

- when used appropriately, only caries-infected dentine is removed; mineralised caries-free dentine is preserved, thereby limiting damage to the pulpal tissues
- avoidance of local anaesthesia and rotary cutting instruments for caries removal, which is of psychological benefit to certain patients.

The main disadvantage of chemomechanical techniques is that they take longer to perform than traditional techniques, thereby requiring increased chair-side time. There is little evidence to demonstrate that the outcome of treatment is different to that obtained with traditional mechanical techniques, except for a reduced risk of iatrogenic damage to adjacent soft tissues and teeth. Increased chair-side time would appear to be the main factor preventing more widespread use of chemomechanical techniques.

Other Approaches to Caries Management

"Non-traditional" and novel approaches to caries management include, amongst others, the application of ozone delivered as a gas to caries. However, in the absence of good-quality evidence, the efficacy of ozone treatments in managing caries remains equivocal.

Cavity Preparation: Promising Approaches

Amongst promising new methods of shaping cavities prior to restoration placement, special mention should be made of sonic techniques. Sonic handpieces have been developed together with interchangeable tips. An example of such a system is SONICflex (KaVo Dental). Sonic instruments facilitate minimally interventive dentistry while minimising trauma to dentine. "Safe-sided" tips limit damage to adjacent soft tissues and teeth during proximal cavity preparations, with limited heat generation. The use of such instrumentation may be facilitated by using traditional rotary instrumentation to make the initial penetration of enamel to provide access to underlying caries. Other new technologies include the use of bioactive glasses in novel air-abrasion methodologies. The selective removal of carious tooth tissue offers excellent opportunities for minimally interventive operative dentistry.

44

Cavity Isolation: No Substitute for Good Technique
Intuitively, we know that effective moisture control is essential when placing any restoration, including posterior composites. Given the hydrophobic nature of composite resins and bonding agents, such materials are moisture sensitive. This becomes a challenge when restoring posterior teeth. Some strategies to overcome this challenge include the use of:
• rubber dam
• other moisture control devices, such as cotton wool rolls, gauze, and dry guards
• close support dentistry aided by high-volume aspiration, effective soft tissue retraction and skilled use of a three-in-one syringe.

Historically, it was thought that the use of rubber dam was essential for the successful placement of posterior composite resin restorations. The advantages of rubber dam include:
• excellent means of moisture control
• patient comfort
• reduced microbial contamination of prepared cavities
• effective infection control through elimination of salivary splatter and aerosols
• elimination of the risk of inhalation of materials and debris, let alone small items of instrumentation.

Surveys of the use of rubber dam in general dental practice indicate, however, that many practitioners choose not to use it, despite its many advantages. Interestingly, while surveys of rubber dam usage report that dentists do not use it as they feel that "patients don't like it", surveys of patients attitudes to rubber dam reveal the opposite. Notwithstanding such considerations, recent studies have demonstrated that the use of rubber dam during the placement of posterior composites does not necessarily lead to increased longevity. It is the quality of the moisture control achieved during placement, rather than the means of control, that is critical. Poor moisture control, whether it be through ineffective rubber dam placement or the inappropriate use of alternative methods, will compromise both the initial quality and the subsequent clinical performance of posterior composites.

Whichever moisture-control technique is used, attention to detail is critical. If moisture contamination occurs, it cannot be ignored.

How is rubber dam placed?
The rubber dam armamentarium (Fig 4-14) consists of:

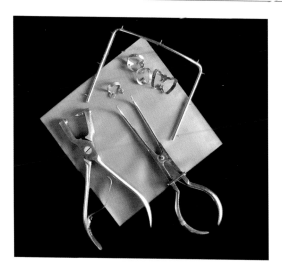

Fig 4-14 The rubber dam armamentarium.

- rubber dam, of appropriate weight (thickness) for the intended purpose
- rubber dam punch, which must be capable of cleanly cutting the rubber dam material
- rubber dam clamps, in a variety of sizes and patterns to cover at least all the common sizes and shapes of tooth
- auxiliary forms of rubber dam retention, including rubber wedges and dental floss
- rubber dam forceps, appropriate for the preferred types of clamp
- rubber dam frames, to stabilise and retract the rubber dam during the operative procedure.

When placing rubber dam, it is first necessary to identify the number of teeth to be isolated, as well as the tooth that will be clamped to retain the rubber dam. For operative procedures, including the placement of posterior composites, a number of teeth should be isolated to give good access to the operating site. The tooth selected to retain the rubber dam clamp is usually the most posterior of the teeth isolated, though difficulties will be encountered if this tooth is to be restored with the aid of a matrix.

Using the rubber dam punch, a series of holes are created in the rubber dam; these should:
- be situated in the centre of the rubber dam sheet, rather along an edge
- follow a curved orientation, similar to the arrangement of the teeth to be isolated

- be adequately spaced to ensure that an appropriate amount of rubber dam is present in the proximal contact areas
- be of appropriate size and cleanly cut to limit the risk of the dam tearing when stretched.

An appropriate clamp should be selected. The choice of a winged or a non-winged clamp is a matter of clinical preference, but generally it is felt that a winged clamp is more retentive. For safety reasons, dental floss should be tied to the rubber dam clamp to facilitate rescue of the clamp should it be accidentally swallowed or inhaled.

The exact sequence of placing the various components of the rubber dam is a matter of clinical preference. Possible techniques include:
- the placement of the clamp to the selected tooth, followed by the rubber dam, which is stretched to pass over the clamped tooth
- the placement of the rubber dam over the selected teeth, followed by rubber dam clamp placement
- the rubber dam and clamp are applied simultaneously.

It may be helpful to apply lubricant to the rubber dam to facilitate placement, but the lubricant must not contaminate the eventual cavity preparation. Whichever technique is used, the help of a suitably trained chair-side assistant, ideally a dental nurse, will facilitate rapid and effective placement of the dam.

The rubber dam frame may be applied simultaneously or following rubber dam placement. Care should be taken to ensure that the rubber dam frame does not cause trauma to the patient's lips, cheeks or face. The rubber dam itself may sometimes need to be modified to allow the patient to breathe comfortably.

Cavity Design Features

The cavity design features for posterior composite restorations are very different to those for dental amalgam restorations. Cavity design for posterior dental amalgam restorations is often determined by materials considerations. For example, a 2 mm thickness of dental amalgam is required to optimise the physical properties of the restoration. Other design features of cavities for posterior dental amalgam restorations include:
- sacrifice of significant amounts of intact and healthy tooth tissue to provide mechanical retention and resistance form
- removal of occlusal tooth tissue to create occlusal "locks" or "dovetails" to help to provide retention for occlusoproximal restorations

- the incorporation of well-defined internal line and point angles. These will effectively concentrate forces at the base of cavities, potentially leading in the long term to fracture.

In contrast, cavity design for posterior composite restorations is largely determined by the location and extent of the caries. Modern composite resin materials and associated bonding technologies have now reached a level of sophistication that it is often sufficient simply to remove dentine that has been irreversibly damaged and heavily infected by caries, and then to place an adhesive composite restoration to restore fully form, function and appearance.

As composite restorations are adhesive, and there is no need to remove intact tooth substance to create mechanical undercuts, the benefits for the lifelong preservation of the tooth are evident (Fig 4-15).

Some specific design features that should be considered when planning to restore a posterior tooth with composite resin include:
- access, sufficient to see and remove irreversibly damaged dentine
- the incorporation of rounded internal line angles
- the placement of margins away from occlusal contacts
- carefully finished cavosurface margins, possibly including intra-enamel bevels but not long low-surface bevels.

Access is critical for the successful removal of irreversibly damaged dentine and for the subsequent placement of composite. Lack of access, as occurs in tunnel preparations, is considered to be the downfall of ultraconservative cavity designs, which are theoretically attractive but practically ineffective.

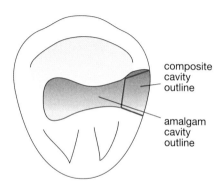

composite
cavity
outline

amalgam
cavity
outline

Fig 4-15 Differences in cavity design for posterior occlusoproximal dental amalgam and composite resin restorations.

Rounded internal line features (line and point angles) not only save sound dentine but also improve the biomechanical features of the restored tooth. Rounded internal features mean few, if any, damaging high-stress points are incorporated into the restoration; such stress points can lead to catastrophic failure, including cuspal fracture.

The placement of occlusal margins away from occlusal contacts will extend the longevity of the restoration by helping to preserve marginal integrity. The presence and location of occlusal contacts should be assessed when the cavity outlined is being planned, importantly prior to rubber dam placement. While the outline of the cavity should be conservative, it may need to be extended to leave margins away from occlusal contacts. Alternatively, and where possible, occlusal contacts may be adjusted to preserve enamel. One of the aims of the design of the occlusal outline is to preserve enamel-to-enamel contacts.

Finally, while it is appropriate to place long low bevels on the cavosurface margins of anterior cavities prior to placing composite restorations, this is inappropriate in cavities for posterior composites (Figs 4-16 and 4-17). Bevelling of occlusal cavosurface margins will lead to thin extensions of composite resin on the occlusal surface. Such thin extensions will either fracture under occlusal loading or lead to unnecessary enlargement of the cavity at the time of any subsequent operative intervention. Bevelling of the proximal cavosurface margin causes unnecessary loss of valuable enamel, but more importantly it will lead to substantial marginal excesses below the contact area. Such excesses are very difficult to remove without causing a great deal of iatrogenic damage.

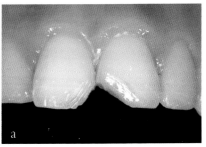 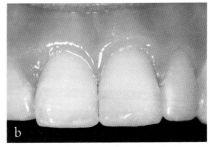

Fig 4-16 When placing an anterior composite restoration, long low bevels should be placed along the anterior cavosurface margin. The incorporation of such bevels (a) permits a smooth, imperceptible transition between composite restoration and natural tooth (b). (Restoration made in Miris 2, Coltène Whaledent, Switzerland.)

49

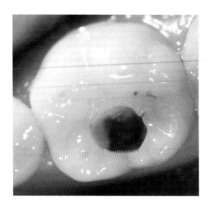

Fig 4-17 Completed cavity preparation for posterior composite restoration. Notice the absence of long low bevels on the cavosurface margins (this is a replacement restoration, the shape of the cavity being determined by the previous restoration).

In summary, cavity design for posterior composite restorations is distinctly different to that for dental amalgam restorations and is determined in the main by the location, nature and extent of the caries.

Key Learning Points

- The changing patterns of dental disease, notably caries, challenges the diagnostic and technical skills of dental practitioners.
- Increasingly, the approach to the management of caries should follow a minimally interventive biological approach. New methods of caries diagnosis and instrumentation for cavity preparation can facilitate this approach.
- Moisture control is essential when placing posterior composite restorations, though the placement of rubber dam is not always required for this purpose.
- The design features of posterior cavities prepared for placement of composite resin is very different to those prepared for dental amalgam restorations.

Further Reading

Brunthaler A, Konig F, Lucas T, Sperr W, Schedle A. Longevity of direct resin composite restorations in posterior teeth. Clin Oral Invest 2003;7:63–70.

Lynch CD, McConnell RJ. Attitudes and use of rubber dam by Irish general dental practitioners. Int Endod J 2007;40:427–432.

Wilson NHF. Minimally Invasive Dentistry. London: Quintessence, 2007.

Chapter 5
Protecting Dentine and Pulp: Do We Really Need a Base?

Aim

The aim of this chapter is to describe and review the various techniques available for protecting dentine and pulp prior to the placement of posterior composite restorations.

Outcome

At the end of this chapter, the reader will:
- appreciate why the protection of dentine and pulp is necessary when restoring posterior teeth
- understand how the philosophy of protecting dentine and pulp has changed in recent years
- appreciate the range of techniques available for protecting dentine and pulp prior to the placement of posterior composite restorations.

Introduction

On completion of caries removal, operatively exposed dentine must be assessed and managed in a careful and judicious manner to avoid subsequent pulpal irritation or death. All dentine should be regarded as "vital" tissue in intimate communication with the dental pulp. The density of dentinal tubules in coronal human dentine is reported in Table 5-1. Even shallow cavities involving dentine may contain dentinal tubules up to a density of $8,000/mm^2$ in cuspal regions.

The most common cause of pulpal damage and death is bacterial contamination. Such contamination can be a consequence of a failure to manage dentine caries subsequent to leakage of a deficient or inadequately sealed restoration. A further cause of pulpal damage is trauma, either in the form of a blow to the tooth, with or without a fracture, or much more commonly iatrogenic trauma from dental instrumentation. A more subtle, though no less critical, consideration is the manner in which operatively exposed dentine is handled. As already emphasised, dentine is a "live" tissue (in contrast to "dead"

Table 5-1 **Distribution of dentinal tubules within human coronal dentine**

Level	Distribution (per mm²)			
	Occlusal	Cuspal	Middle crown	Cemento-enamel junction
Outer	8,000	20,000	10,000	10,000
Middle	32,000	36,000	32,000	29,000
Inner	58,000	58,000	48,000	48,000

Source: Mjör & Nordahl, 1996.

enamel). It is moist, wet, capable of autorepair and in direct communication with the pulp. As such, it can be "insulted" or damaged by the injudicious use of dull burs, aggressive cutting actions, inadequate water cooling during mechanical preparation, and continuous rather than intermittent cutting (Fig 5-1). Dentine needs to be managed with great care at all times.

It was once thought that contact between certain restorative materials and dentine, or failure to thermally insulate a cavity were events capable of causing pulpal death. It is now widely accepted that the effects of restorative materials on the pulp are transitory, and the pulp seems to be far more capable of withstanding intraoral changes in temperature than was previously thought.

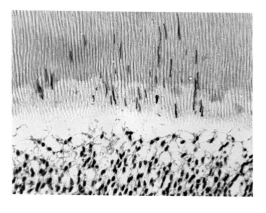

Fig 5-1 An example of trauma to the pulp–dentine complex during aggressive cavity preparation; this stained histological image taken from a canine tooth shows odontoblasts (stained purple) that have been displaced into dentinal tubules following aggressive cutting actions in a deep dentinal cavity. (Courtesy of Professor VR O'Sullivan, Royal College of Surgeons in Ireland – Medical University of Bahrain.)

It follows, therefore, that the primary consideration following caries removal is the protection of the pulp from immediate or subsequent bacterial contamination. This challenge is greatest when the pulp has been exposed.

Management of Exposed Pulpal Tissues

Dental pulp is a complex tissue containing blood vessels, nerves and cells, including odontoblasts. Odontoblastic processes and numerous nerve fibres extend from the pulp into the dentine, making the dentine vital and sensitive to stimuli (Fig 5-2). When exposed to the effects of the carious process, or repeated stimuli, the pulpal odontoblasts are capable of producing further hard dentinal tissue, variously referred to as "sclerotic", "reactionary", "reparative" or "tertiary" dentine. This reaction is intended to distance the pulp from the caries and other stimuli, and in the process protect the pulp from bacterial contamination. In the presence of active, rapidly advancing caries and atypical stimuli, the defences of the pulpodentinal complex may be overwhelmed, with subsequent death of the pulp.

When dealing with an exposed pulp that has suffered reversible rather than irreversible damage, it is necessary to make certain clinical judgements on the most appropriate management. Such judgements should be based on a risk assessment. Before commencing treatment, the extent of a deep, penetrating lesion of caries should be assessed radiographically. In accordance

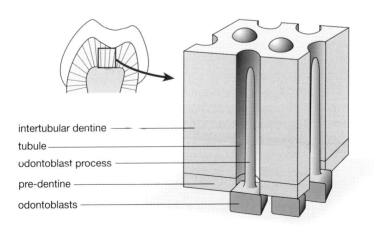

intertubular dentine

tubule

odontoblast process

pre-dentine

odontoblasts

Fig 5-2 Schematic diagram of the intimate contact between pulp and dentine.

with good practice, clinical and radiographic assessment should be accompanied by vitality testing, transillumination and other diagnostic tests as may be indicated clinically (Fig 5-3).

The management of an operatively exposed pulp depends on three main factors:
• the size of the pulpal exposure
• the extent and persistence of pulpal bleeding
• the nature and extent of caries adjacent to the exposure.

The most significant factor in pulpal inflammation and death is the presence of bacteria. Clearly, if the caries extends to the pulp, then the pulp must be considered to be infected and, in all probability, irretrievably damaged. If, however, the caries has not reached the pulp, then it may be possible to stimulate pulpal healing and formation of a hard-tissue barrier using a direct pulp-capping technique. Materials recommended for this procedure include hard fast-setting calcium hydroxide cements and, more recently, mineral trioxide aggregate (MTA). Good isolation is paramount when managing a direct pulpal exposure in order to minimise bacterial contamination. If rubber dam has not already been applied (a good prophylactic measure if caries is diagnosed preoperatively to be deep and potentially close to the pulp), then the few minutes necessary to apply it is time well spent. Needless to say, if attempts to apply a rubber dam are anticipated to result in the cavity being awash with saliva, then immediate isolation with cotton wool rolls, supported as appropriate by salivary ejectors, is to be favoured. While direct pulp-capping techniques have an acceptable success rate, there is still a risk of pulpal death in the medium to long term, necessitating subsequent monitoring of pulp vitality.

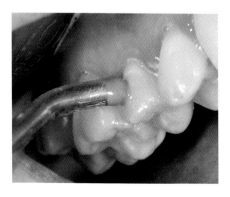

Fig 5-3 Vitality testing of a maxillary second premolar using an electric pulp tester.

When a direct pulp cap has been placed, it is important to protect it with a glass–ionomer cement (GIC) base. To be effective, such a base must be at least 0.5 mm thick. Furthermore, to preclude the possibility of leakage, the GIC base should not be excessively air dried or otherwise dehydrated.

The size and extent of the pulpal exposure is important. Large (> 0.5 mm) pulpal exposures are more likely to lead to pulp death than small exposures. Accordingly, the extent of the pulpal exposure should be recorded in the patient's clinical records. The extent of pulpal bleeding may indicate the extent of any pulpal inflammation present, but assessments of bleeding can be very subjective and are, therefore, poor indicators of pulp prognosis. Failure to control pulpal bleeding prior to pulp capping will compromise the prognosis of the pulp. In situations in which there is limited (< 0.5 mm) remaining dentinal thickness over the pulp, but all the grossly softened and infected caries has been removed, an indirect pulp-capping technique may be employed. Fast hard-setting calcium hydroxide cements have been recommended for this purpose. However, it is very difficult to determine the thickness of dentine remaining over the pulp, in particular to a sensitivity of 0.5 mm. Indications of the need for an indirect pulp cap include proximity of caries to the pulp on radiographic examination and a pinkish hue to the base of the cavity.

To Base or not to Base …

Much of the traditional thinking regarding the management of operatively exposed dentine in posterior teeth is based on the use of dental amalgam. As dental amalgam is thermo- and electroconductive, it was considered necessary to place a cement base to provide insulation, thereby protecting the pulp from repeated damaging insults. Notwithstanding the fact that the evidence base for such techniques was limited, this management approach has been carried over into techniques for the placement of posterior composites, more to protect the pulp from alleged adverse effects of resin-based materials than from thermal, let alone electrical, stimuli. It is now known that:

- the use of a base, in particular a thick base (> 1.5 mm), can lead to an overall reduction in the strength of the restored tooth unit, let alone the restoration
- appropriately placed and polymerised composites do not have significant adverse effects on the underlying pulp and, consequently, do not need to be separated from the pulp by a base
- a composite with an effective marginal seal is not dependent on an underlying base to protect the pulp from the damaging adverse effects of bacteria.

Each of these considerations, together with the development of increasingly predictable and sophisticated dentine bonding systems, has led many to question the value of placing a base under a composite restoration. Some clinicians now prefer to utilise only a dentine bonding system to seal and protect the underlying dentine and pulp.

Considerable confusion exists regarding the management of operatively exposed dentine in the middle and inner regions of the tooth. There is almost universal agreement that shallow cavities to be restored with composite are best managed by etching and bonding alone. However, when managing cavities extending into the middle and inner thirds of dentine, surveys of techniques used by general dental practitioners, as well as surveys of current teaching, have indicated that there is great variation in both the techniques used in general practice and those taught in dental schools. This variation is a reflection of the lack of appropriate evidence with respect to the management of operatively exposed dentine. With this in mind, the clinical techniques described in the rest of this chapter for dentinal and pulpal protection are based on current best-available evidence.

Sticking With What We Know: Bases

As discussed in the previous section, cement bases were used historically to prevent repeated adverse stimulation of the underlying dentine and pulp subjacent to dental amalgam or other metallic restorations. The materials used included zinc phosphate and zinc oxide and eugenol cements. With the introduction of GICs and the subsequent development of resin-modified GICs (RMGICs), zinc phosphate and zinc oxide and eugenol cements were progressively replaced. GIC systems having the major advantage of adhesion to the underlying dentine.

Glass–ionomer Systems

The GICs are the only group of restorative dental materials capable of true auto-adherence to dentine. The setting reactions of GICs are based on an aqueous acid–base mechanism. This water-based chemistry makes GICs more moisture friendly, and less technique sensitive than, for example, composite resins. The adhesion mechanism for GICs is developed in two ways:
- the formation of an interlocking interface between the GIC and dentine: micromechanical retention
- the formation of ionic bonds between carboxyl groups in the GICs and calcium molecules in the surface of the exposed dentine: chemical bonding.

These mechanisms, in addition to providing retention, create an interfacial seal between the GIC and dentine, limiting the ingress of bacteria and, in turn, the risk of pulpal irritation.

As GICs are mildly acidic, there is an element of "self-etching" involved in the adhesive process. To assist this process, it is sometimes useful also to apply a weak conditioner to the prepared dentinal surfaces to enhance adhesion. This is especially helpful when a great deal of debris and smear has been created during cavity preparation, as occurs when coarse-cutting diamond burs have been used. The application of such a conditioner will remove the smear layer, exposing the underlying dentine, and allow better wetting of the surface and enhanced adhesion.

The release of fluoride from GICs has been argued to have cariostatic or even anticariogenic properties. There is, however, little evidence to support such effects in clinical service.

Possible concerns regarding the use of GICs as a base material include:
- they do not form a rigid base, possibly predisposing the overlying restoration to fracture under heavy occlusal loading
- as the setting chemistry is water based, they are at some risk of "dissolution" if they become exposed to oral fluids
- given the nature of the acid–base setting reaction of GICs, bases of these materials are not fully set at the time of restoration placement.

Resin-modified Glass–ionomers
To counter the limitations of traditional GICs, the RMGICs were developed. These cements are, at their simplest, GICs to which a resin phase has been added. Typically the GIC:resin ratio is of the order of 4:1. The inclusion of the resin phase has advantages. These advantages include:
- increased compressive strengths and a reduced tendency to brittle fracture
- increased wear resistance
- increased resistance to dissolution in oral fluids
- capacity to be "command set" through dual cure mechanisms.

The use of RMGICs is now recommended over traditional GICs for basing cavities. When used as a base, the resin phase of RMGICs can be light activated and command set, allowing immediate placement of the restoration. The acid–base setting reaction of the GIC element of the RMGIC continues for some time subsequent to restoration placement.

57

The advantages of using adhesive bases of, in particular, the RMGIC systems include the ability to:
• prevent bacterial leakage along the tooth–base interface
• bond to an adhesively retained restoration
• avoid the need to resort to the outmoded and outdated approach of using dentinal pins to help to retain the restoration.

Clinically, bases may be:
• applied in bulk, in situations in which the base is being used to replace lost dentine
• applied in a relatively thin (> 0.5 mm) layer to protect an indirect or direct pulp cap of a material such as a hard-setting calcium hydroxide cement.

The use of a "bulk" base limits the thickness of the overlying restoration. A reduction in the thickness of a restoration reduces fracture resistance. Furthermore, the use of a "bulk base" will reduce the surface area of dentine available for bonding. Given such considerations, let alone the lack of long-term clinical evidence demonstrating superior clinical outcomes with "bulk" bases, the rationale for their use is increasingly questioned, in particular when placing adhesively bonded posterior composites (Fig 5-4).

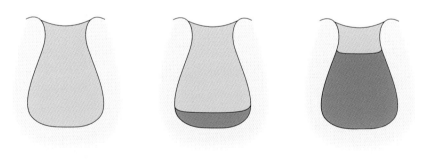

No base
• maximal area for bonding
• maximal thickness of composite

Thin base
• area for bonding ↓
• thickness of composite ↓

Bulk base
• minimal area for bonding
• minimal thickness of composite

Fig 5-4 Schematic diagram illustrating the differences between "bulk" and "thin" bases.

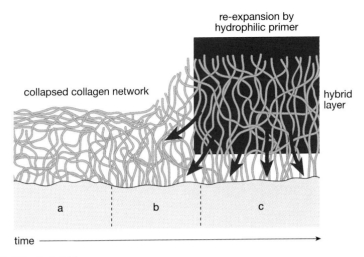

re-expansion by
hydrophilic primer

collapsed collagen network

hybrid
layer

a   b   c

time

Fig 5-5 The hybrid layer.

New Approaches

Given the limitations associated with "bulk" bases under posterior composite restorations, what alternative strategies are available? One obvious possibility is the use of dentine-bonding agents only. As described in Chapter 2, predictable and satisfactory dentine bonding is now a reality in clinical dentistry. Dentine-bonding agents are commercially available as both "etch and rinse" (three-step and two-step) and "self-etching" (two-step and one-step) application systems. These adhesive mechanisms have the clinical advantages of:

- retention by means of micromechanical interlocking, including the formation of a hybrid layer with the exposed dentinal collagenous network and accessible dentinal tubules (Fig 5-5)
- a marginal seal, thus protecting the underlying dentine and pulp from bacterial microleakage
- avoidance of the use of dentine pins, with their associated stresses within the tooth
- avoidance of the use of a base, optimising the mechanical properties of the completed restoration.

Assuming good marginal integrity, the dentinal tubules can effectively be "sealed" from potentially pathogenic bacteria. Though no long-term clinical evidence exists to support the use of dentine-bonding agents in preference to RMGICs/GICs, the use of dentine-bonding agents simplifies the placement of the restoration (thereby reducing the risk of operator error) and enhances the biomechanics of the restored tooth unit. It could, therefore, be argued that dentine-bonding agents should be used in preference to bases in all situations. There are, however, certain situations that require special attention. These include:

• providing protection for a direct or indirect pulp cap of a hard-setting calcium hydroxide, which would be damaged by the direct application of an acid etchant or self-etching primer/bonding system
• where obtaining an adequate marginal seal may be difficult, for example a subgingival margin in a proximal restoration.

The latter situation presents a particular challenge. It is often difficult to achieve a marginal seal where the cavity extends subgingivally, given the proposed composite restoration finishing on dentine and cementum, let alone the difficulties of moisture control. Such an environment is clearly not "composite-friendly", and as such, the marginal integrity of any composite restoration placed in such circumstances will be dubious. A way to overcome this difficulty is to restore the subgingival region of the cavity using a base of RMGIC. The composite restoration can then be placed with relatively little, if any, risk of moisture contamination. This combined use of materials is referred to as an "open sandwich". Relatively good success has been reported with this technique when RMGICs have been used. Traditional GICs should be avoided in these scenarios as they tend to "wash-out", with subsequent post-operative sensitivity and the development of secondary caries.

As will be discussed in Chapter 6, some practitioners like to place a flowable composite resin (with a low filler:resin ratio) as an "elastic" base for posterior composite restorations; it is thought this technique introduces a degree of "stress breaking" or stress dissipation during polymerisation, thereby avoiding flexure, or "stressing", of opposing cusps or cavity walls. Notwithstanding the recognised limitations of flowable composites, such as excessive contraction and the incorporation of excessive polymerisation stresses, there is little good long-term clinical evidence to support this technique. Polymerisation stresses are best managed by careful incremental placement.

Some final considerations regarding protection for dentine and pulp are as follows.

• Prior to placement of a dentine-bonding agent, caution should always be exercised when etching dentine. When phosphoric acid is being used, dentine should be etched for only 15 seconds (Figs 5-6 to 5-9).

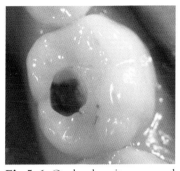

Fig 5-6 Occlusal cavity prepared in a mandibular first molar.

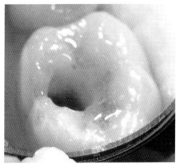

Fig 5-7 Phosphoric acid etchant applied to the enamel alone for 30 seconds.

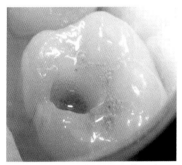

Fig 5-8 Phosphoric acid etchant then applied to both dentine and enamel for remaining 15 seconds.

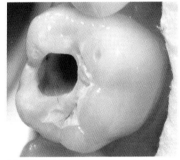

Fig 5-9 The enamel and dentine are dried gently. A "frosted" appearance develops on the enamel, while the dentine maintains a "moist" appearance.

Prolonged etching, let alone excessive drying, can give rise to sustained post-treatment sensitivity.

- While there is no evidence that rubber dam isolation is essential, there is no question that a well-placed rubber dam greatly facilitates the placement of a posterior composite, including effective bonding.
- Dentine bonding systems are very technique sensitive. Furthermore, even well-placed dentine adhesives may suffer some leakage and, in time, hydrolytic degeneration. Dentine bonding is, therefore, a procedure to be undertaken with great care and attention, let alone strict compliance with the manufacturer's directions for use.

Key Learning Points

- Dentine and pulpal protection is a significant clinical consideration when placing restorations, including posterior composite restorations.
- The use of adhesive restorations avoids the use of dentine pins, which can incorporate stress into the underlying tooth structure.
- Dentine can be protected by the use of RMGIC bases or a dentine-bonding agent.
- If used to best advantage, dentine-bonding agents offer effective retention, marginal seal and favourable biomechanical features in the completed restoration.
- There is no long-term clinical evidence to support the placement of flowable composite resins as a liner under posterior composite restorations.
- Dentine-bonding agents are only as good as the technique used to place them.

Reference

Mjör IA, Nordahl I. The density and branching of dentinal tubules in human teeth. Arch Oral Biol 1996;41:401–412.

Further Reading

Burke FM, McConnell RJ, Ray NJ. Fluoride-containing restorative materials. Int Dent J 2006;56:33–43.

Lynch CD, McConnell RJ, Wilson NHF. Trends in the placement of posterior composites in dental schools. J Dent Educ 2007;71:430–434.

van Meerbeek B, de Munck J, Yoshida Y, Inoue S, Vargas M, Vijay P, van Landuyt K, Lambrechts P, Vanherle G. Adhesion to enamel and dentin: current status and future challenges. Oper Dent 2003;28:215–235.

Chapter 6

Shedding Light on Placement Techniques for Posterior Composites

Aim

The aim of this chapter is to describe and review the various techniques available for placing composite resin restorations in load-bearing cavities in posterior teeth.

Outcome

At the end of this chapter, the reader will:
- be aware of the need for adequate moisture control when placing posterior composite restorations
- have knowledge of the various techniques available for restoring load-bearing cavities in posterior teeth using composite resin
- understand the need for appropriate placement techniques, such as incremental layering and selection of appropriate light-curing techniques.

Introduction

Historically, many of the problems associated with the use of composite resin in posterior teeth, such as persistent post-treatment sensitivity, loss of retention and secondary caries, were caused by inappropriate material selection and placement techniques. As has been discussed, there are some basic principles that must always be adhered to when placing posterior composites:
- composite resin is not "tooth-coloured" silver amalgam and, as such, cannot be handled in the same way as silver amalgam; notably attempts should not be made to condense a composite resin into a cavity
- composite resin should be adapted, sculpted and shaped to the internal features of the cavity
- composite resin should not be bulk placed or bulk polymerised in any cavity, including those in posterior teeth
- careful consideration must be given to material selection to ensure that the completed restoration can withstand repeated occlusal loading, while still presenting an aesthetic appearance (Chapter 2).

The range of clinical situations in which composite resin restorations will function satisfactorily is ever expanding. This success is a reflection of a greater understanding of, and careful attention to, composite placement techniques, along with the improvement in quality and sophistication of composite resin materials and associated bonding technologies.

Isolation

As discussed in Chapter 4, adequate moisture control is essential when placing posterior composite restorations. A wet environment is clearly not compatible with the hydrophobic nature of composite resin materials and associated bonding technologies. Placement of a rubber dam is not, however, always necessary prior to placement of a composite restoration. According to best available evidence, the longevity of posterior composite restorations placed with high-quality moisture control, for example using high-volume aspiration and cotton wool rolls, is comparable to the longevity of those placed under rubber dam. While the rubber dam may provide a clear operating field, with good access for placement of composite resin material, and prevent potentially harmful agents such as phosphoric acid coming into contact with soft tissues, its use is not critical to the survival of restorations. It is the quality of the isolation that matters, not the technique used to achieve it.

Placement

At this stage of providing a posterior composite restoration, the cavity has been prepared (Chapter 4), and the dentine has been protected in an appropriate manner (Chapter 5). What happens next depends on the nature of composite resin to be placed. To understand this, it is necessary to consider the clinically relevant properties of composite resin materials, including:
• the significance of the filler:resin ratio
• polymerisation contraction and polymerisation stress
• the polymerisation mechanism: light activation chemistry and depth of cure
• curing time.

The Significance of the Filler:Resin Ratio
As described in Chapter 2, composite resins are a mixture of a plastic resin, usually bisphenol A glycidyl methacrylate (bis-GMA), and filler particles (usually silica), which are linked using a coupling agent. The physical properties of the composite resin material selected are a reflection of the filler particle size and the filler content of the material. Given the varied demands

placed on anterior and posterior composite restorations, there is, as yet, no composite resin material that can be truly described as a "universal" material suitable for both anterior and posterior use. Posterior cavities require composite resin material with high filler:resin ratio when considered by volume, not by weight (as discussed in Chapter 2, consideration of the filler:resin ratio by weight does not have the same implications for the physical properties of the material as consideration by volume). Such materials, being of relatively high-compressive strength, high-wear resistance and acceptable aesthetic qualities, are suited to posterior cavities but cannot be recommended for anterior cavities. Given the amount and size of filler particles in composites with high filler:resin ratios, restorations of these materials cannot be polished to the extent necessary to produce a suitably "aesthetic" anterior restoration; they also have a relatively opaque appearance. Composite resin materials that contain a filler:resin ratio in excess of 60% are suitable for restoring posterior load-bearing cavities. Conversely, resins best suited for use in anterior teeth should not be placed in posterior cavities, where relatively low filler:resin ratios would result in increased wear and ultimate failure under compressive occlusal loading.

Polymerisation Contraction and Polymerisation Stress

A significant property of composite resin materials that must be considered when planning a restoration is polymerisation contraction (shrinkage). The resin component of composite resin in its unpolymerised, or uncured, state consists of many small chains of low molecular weight, referred to as monomers. When polymerisation is initiated, these activated monomer units join together to form polymers, or longer molecular chains. In the early stages of the polymerisation process, the material enters a "gel" stage, where linkages are being formed but the material is still relatively soft. The transformation from the gel stage to the final polymerised state is associated with the occurrence of polymerisation stresses within the material and an overall contraction in the mass of the composite resin material. The overall degree of contraction is related to the filler:resin ratio and the dimensions of the composite material being cured at any one time. Materials with a relatively low filler:resin ratio contract more than those with a greater filler:resin ratio. As the former contains proportionately more resin, polymerising larger amounts of this material will lead to more polymerisation contraction than would occur when smaller amounts of the same material are polymerised.

While shrinkage of composite resin material is unavoidable, usually in the order of 2–3%, techniques should be used to limit the effects of the contraction. Clinically, this means that bulk curing of a large amount of composite resin is to be avoided. Such an approach could lead to the formation of a marginal gap through which bacteria will gain entry to the base of the cavity.

Alternatively, if the composite remains bonded to the walls of the cavity, the polymerisation contraction will cause the cusps to flex. "Stressed cusps" tend to give rise to post-operative pain, cracking of enamel and may ultimately lead to cuspal fracture. Clearly, placement and curing of composite resin "in bulk" is inappropriate, and an alternative placement strategy must be used. Current opinion and evidence suggests that optimal results are achieved when increments of composite resin are placed, forming oblique layers between a cusp and the base of the cavity rather than linking opposing cusps (Figs 6-1 and 6-2).

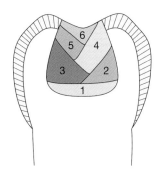

Fig 6-1 An oblique incremental layering technique. (Courtesy of P Brunton, *Decision-making in Operative Dentistry*. London: Quintessence, 2002.)

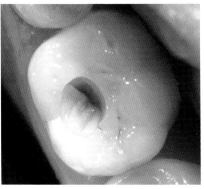

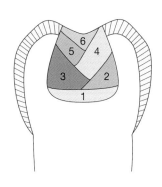

Fig 6-2 Clinical placement of oblique increments.

Polymerisation contraction can also have significant clinical effects in the placement of proximal composite restorations. If the polymerisation contraction is not "factored in" to the clinical technique, it is more difficult to restore the proximal contact. The clinical consequences of a light, let alone open, contact will be familiar to readers, notably proximal food packing, causing pain and, if not corrected, secondary caries and the initiation or progression of periodontal disease. Strategies for managing polymerisation contraction in proximal restorations are described in Chapter 7.

Consideration must also be given to the direction in which polymerisation contraction of composite materials takes place. Previously, it was considered that composite materials contracted in the direction of the incident curing light. This was part of the rationale for the introduction of transparent matrix bands and light-transmitting proximal wedge systems. It was thought that metal matrix bands limited access of the incident curing light, in particular to the base of the proximal box, causing composite covering the gingival seat to "shrink" in an occlusal direction and "lift" away from the base. It is now known that this concept is incorrect; composite materials contract on polymerisation towards the area of "greater adhesion", for example away from dentine towards the overlying enamel (the so-called C-factor). An incremental layering and curing technique, which avoids such polymerisation effects, helps to limit the risk of gap formation or stressed cusps. Given the above, transparent matrix bands and light-transmitting proximal wedges are no longer recommended for use in the placement of proximal posterior composites.

Recently, some consideration has been given to the usefulness of incorporating an "elastic" or "stress-breaking" liner or base under posterior composite restorations as a means of reducing polymerisation stresses. The rationale for using such a liner or base is to accommodate relatively minor movement of opposing cusps and cavity walls during polymerisation, thereby reducing polymerisation stresses. A number of materials and placement techniques have been suggested for achieving this, including:

- placement of a resin–modified glass–ionomer cement base, which should not be light cured; as the acid–base setting reaction proceeds, it is thought that the elastic nature of the setting material allows dissipation of poly-merisation stresses developed in the overlying composite restoration
- placement of a flowable composite resin, with a low filler loading
- the use of a thick-layer bonding agent.

While there is little evidence to support the inclusion of a "stress-breaking" base, let alone the selection of any one clinical technique, this approach has

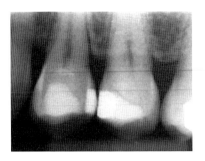

Fig 6-3 The radiolucency underneath the restoration in the maxillary second premolar could be confused with the presentation of caries; it indicates a thick-layer dentine bonding has been used to retain the composite restoration.

had certain popularity amongst clinicians. In light of the discussion in Chapter 5, and the trend to avoid the use of a base under a composite restoration, the use of a resin-modified glass–ionomer cement is not recommended. As discussed elsewhere in this text, the use of a flowable composite resin as a stress breaker is to be avoided, given the degree of polymerisation contraction of such materials and the concomitant incidence of interfacial voids and defects. It is, therefore, suggested that the use of a thick-layer dentine-bonding agent may be the best means of achieving a "stress-breaker" effect. One of the complications of this approach is that bonding agents are radiolucent, and a thick section along a gingival margin may be confused with secondary caries on radiographic examination (Fig 6-3).

The Polymerisation Mechanism

A further consideration in the handling of a composite resin is the means by which the material polymerises. Composite resin, in its unpolymerised state, includes small monomer molecules. These molecules become activated to initiate polymerisation: the formation of long chains of monomer molecules, referred to as polymers.

Broadly, there are two types of activation chemistry for composite resins:
- chemical activation, often referred to as chemical curing: composite resin materials that rely on this form of activation chemistry are usually available as two components, which when mixed together activate polymerisation
- light activation, often referred to as light curing: composite resin materials that rely on this form of activation are available as one component, which is irradiated with light of a specific wavelength to initiate polymerisation.

While chemically cured composite resins materials used to enjoy widespread use, their application in contemporary clinical practice is limited. Some of the reasons for this include a tendency to develop porosity, relatively poor colour stability and the need to wait for these materials to "set" in the mouth. As a consequence, chemically cured composites have been replaced by light-cured materials. This latter group tends to have superior physical properties, less porosity and more colour stability. They also feature the additional advantage of being "command set"; that is, the material, unlike chemically cured composites, is not setting as it is placed, affording good working time, assuming that it is not exposed to sufficient ambient light, in particular from the operating light, to initiate polymerisation.

Light-curing composite resin materials contain a photoinitiator, usually camphoroquinone, which becomes activated to promote production of free-radical molecules when it is irradiated with light of a specific wavelength and appropriate intensity for an appropriate period of time. The free radicals initiate polymerisation, in which individual monomer units join together to form a polymer chain. For a light-cured composite resin material to be fully cured, all of the material should be uniformly exposed to activating light of similar intensity for an appropriate length of time. Intuitively, we know that this is somewhat challenging when restoring a deep or complex occlusal or occlusoproximal cavity in posterior teeth, where the only access for the light source is from the occlusal surface, particularly when a matrix is in place. The shape of the occlusal portion of the cavity can often limit access for light curing, resulting in a reduced intensity of light reaching material "in shadow".

A further complication is that light capable of initiating polymerisation penetrates the semi-opaque material to a limited depth. This property of composite resin materials is referred to as "depth of cure": the depth or thickness of composite resin material through which the activating light can penetrate and effect adequate polymerisation. The clinical importance of depth of cure cannot be overemphasised. If an attempt is made to light cure portions of composite resin in excess of the depth of cure, the regions of material furthest away from the light-curing unit will be inadequately polymerised or possibly even left unpolymerised. Worryingly, this may be difficult to detect clinically, as the surface of the material will be polymerised but deeper regions of the restoration will be inaccessible for inspection. In any case, it is difficult to determine clinically the extent to which a composite restoration has been cured.

Most light-activated composite materials have traditionally included camphoroquinone as a photoinitiator. This material is yellow in colour and problematic in very pale or "bleached" composite shades. While these shades of composite are not commonly used in the placement of posterior composites, readers should be aware that some very pale composites contain alternative photoinitiators with a different absorption spectrum to camphoroquinone, and these may not be adequately cured by all light-curing units.

Curing Times

It is also important that each increment of composite resin material is exposed to incident curing light for an appropriate length of time, usually in the region of 20 to 30 seconds. This is the time it takes for the photoinitiator to be activated. Reducing the curing time tends to result in the early termination of polymerised chains ("short-chain termination"), which, amongst other effects, compromises the mechanical properties of the polymerised material. Rapid curing (short curing times) reduces the time the material remains in the gel stage. The effect of this is to increase polymerisation stresses, reduce mechanical properties and predisposition to premature failure in clinical service. Some curing strategies have been reported to deal with this problem, including "soft-start", "ramped" and "pulsed" curing:

- in **soft-start** curing, sometimes referred to as "stepped" curing, the composite material is first exposed to light of relatively low intensity, followed by an exposure of increased intensity
- in the **ramped** technique, the intensity is increased continuously over the exposure period
- in the **pulsed** technique, sometimes referred to as "pulsed–delayed" curing, a series of exposure pulses are used, each separated by a dark interval.

While it is felt that these techniques increase the length of time the polymerising material remains in its gel stage, hence reducing polymerisation stresses within the restored tooth unit, there is little good evidence to indicate that this influences the clinical performance of posterior composite restorations. It is not often appreciated that light-cured composite restorations continue to polymerise, albeit very slowly, for a period of up to 24 hours following placement. This extended curing does not contraindicate immediate finishing.

Delivering Light Activation

Clearly, the efficacy of a light-curing unit depends on its ability to produce light of suitable wavelength and intensity to ensure the optimal production of free-radical species, thus increasing the likelihood of achieving the best possible polymerisation. The wavelength of light to match the absorption spectrum of camphoroquinone is 470 nm (1 nanometre is 10^{-9} metre or one-thousandth of one thousandth of a millimetre), which is in the blue range of the visible light spectrum. The use of light of this wavelength, with an intensity in the region of 600 mW/cm^2 is sufficient to polymerise an increment of composite resin of not more than 2 mm thickness.

There are now a number of different types of light-curing unit. These include:

• quartz tungsten–halogen (QTH) units
• plasma arc units
• light-emitting diode (LED) units.

Quartz Tungsten–Halogen Units

The QTH is the original form of light-curing unit. It is still the gold standard against which other newer forms of light-curing units are compared. In its simplest form, QTH units contain a "traditional" tungsten filament bulb, which produces light of a wide range of wavelengths; from this all light except that with wavelengths in the region of 470 nm is filtered out. This "exclusion mechanism" includes a "cold-mirror" (a paraboloid dichroic filter) to remove infrared light, a glass filter to remove ultraviolet light, and a blue filter to exclude all other visible light except that of the required wavelength. The light is emitted from the light-curing unit via a light guide in order to deliver the activating light to the desired location. This light guide may be rigid or flexible (Figs 6-4 and 6-5).

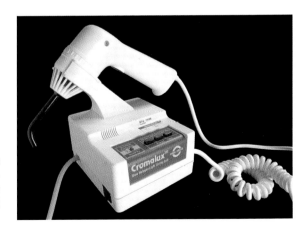

Fig 6-4   A quartz tungsten–halogen light-curing unit. These units are frequently large and bulky.

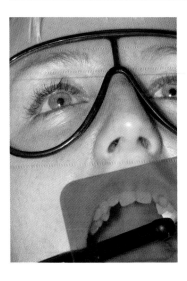

Fig 6-5 The activation light used to initiate polymerisation has the potential to cause retinal damage; therefore, an orange shield should be used to protect the eyes of the operator and assistant.

There are several disadvantages associated with the use of QTH.
• The system is inefficient: extensive filtering of energy in the production of the "blue light" causes heating of the base unit, which needs to be cooled with a fan and can be noisy.
• The performance of QTH bulbs diminishes after a period of possibly as little as six months of regular use; it is impossible to detect this deterioration visually. It can only be determined by using a special electronic device, or light meter. Use of an underperforming QTH will reduce depth of cure of composite, which cannot be detected clinically, and leaves the restoration susceptible to early failure.

In an effort to overcome these disadvantages, newer light-activating technologies have been introduced, with varying degrees of success.

Plasma Arc Lights
Plasma arc lights are based on the application of a high-voltage discharge across two electrodes that are suspended in xenon gas. When the voltage is applied, the gas between the electrodes becomes ionised, creating positively and negatively charged particles. This results in the emission of light of high intensity, usually in the region of 2,500 mW/cm^2, and of a wavelength peaking in the desired region of 470 nm. When plasma arc lights were introduced, it was suggested that they could be used to cure composite materials far more quickly than the traditional QTH unit: light-curing times in the region of

3 seconds were suggested. This was based on the delivery of light of very high intensity. It has transpired, however, that plasma arc lights used in this way are associated with less than ideal clinical outcomes. When compared with QTH units, plasma arc units result in more short-chain termination in polymerised composite. This is associated with reduced physical strength and inferior wear properties: clearly undesirable outcomes when placing, in particular, posterior load-bearing restorations. Polymerisation of composite materials in this fashion is also associated with the generation of high shrinkage stress within the material, ultimately leading to post-operative problems, including sensitivity, cracked tooth syndrome and even catastrophic fracture of the restored tooth unit. Based on such outcomes, the use of plasma arc curing lights tends not to be recommended for the light curing of composite resins.

Light-emitting Diodes

The LED unit is a relatively recent introduction in the field of light-activated composite resin materials. They have, however, shown great promise. The LED unit uses diode technology, incorporating chips containing "doped cells". Electron movement within these cells produces light that matches the absorption spectrum of camphoroquinone. The LED unit has several advantages over QTH units, including:

- more energy efficient, the only light produced is that of the required wavelength
- typically cordless, rechargeable, lightweight, compact and durable
- relatively easy to position and hold in the mouth as they are portable and compact (Fig 6-6a)
- not associated with significant heat generation so remain cool and do not need an integral fan

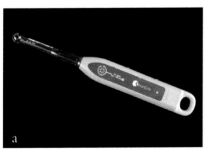
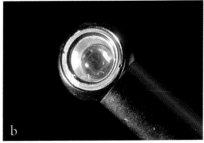

Fig 6-6 A second-generation light-emitting diode (LED) light-curing unit. (a) The device is light and portable, and it can be easily manoeuvred in the oral cavity. (b) There is a single LED chip, which is visible in the centre of the image.

- depth of cure is comparable to, if not greater than, that obtained with the QTH units.

The LED light-curing technology has undergone several refinements subsequent to its introduction. In a similar manner to bonding agents, the term "generation" is used to describe ever more sophisticated units.

- First-generation units consisted of an array of relatively low-powered chips, with low power output and relatively poor curing performance.
- Second-generation units consist of one large chip (Fig 6-6b) and have much more power output than first-generation units. The second-generation LED units have curing performance comparable to that of QTH units. There is, however, some heat generation within these LED units and this may result in "burn-out" of the light-producing chip.
- Third-generation LED units (Fig 6-7) have been designed to avoid heat production and the associated disadvantages. These units also have one high-powered large chip, as used in the second-generation units, but heat production is limited by surrounding it with an array of low-powered smaller chips that produce the required activating light in an alternating sequence.

While satisfactory results have been described with second-generation LED units, there is as yet little information available on the efficacy of third-generation units.

It is also worth remembering that some novel pale and "bleached" shades of composite resin contain alternative photoinitiators to camphoroquinone. The absorption spectrum of these materials, which may occasionally be used

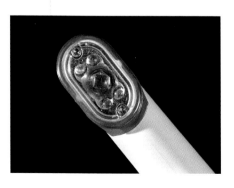

Fig 6-7 In contrast to second-generation light-emitting diode (LED) light-curing units, the newer third-generation units contain a large LED chip (centre of image) and a number of smaller chips surrounding it. These smaller chips produce activating light in sequence, rather than simultaneously.

in placing posterior composites, is not the same as that of camphoroquinone (i.e. not 470 nm). This has caused difficulties with first-, and some second-generation LED units. This has not been a problem with third-generation LED units, or QTH units. Use of a curing unit that produces light which does not match the absorption spectrum of the "alternate" photoinitiator can result in inadequately cured composite restorations.

General Notes on Composite Polymerisation and Placement

It should always be remembered that adequate polymerisation of a composite material is dependent on a number of factors.

- The wavelength and intensity of the curing light: inappropriate wavelengths and intensities are associated with inadequate polymerisation.
- The curing time: inadequate curing times are associated with inadequate polymerisation. As a general rule, curing times should be of the order of 30 seconds for a 2 mm increment of composite. Composite resins do not suffer any adverse effects from extended exposures to curing light; however, care is required with extended exposure to preclude the possibility of adverse heating effects.
- Size, location and orientation of the light guide: direct application of the activating light to the surface of the composite material is associated with optimal polymerisation. Cusps and matrices can limit the approximation of the light guide to the material being cured; similarly in deep cavities, the light guide cannot be approximated to the material being cured. In such circumstances, the thickness of the increment of composite being cured should be reduced and extended exposure times to the light may be indicated.
- Shade of the material: material of a dark shade needs to be cured for longer periods of time or to be placed and cured in relatively thin increments.
- Thickness of the material: composite material should be cured in increments of 2 mm or less to ensure adequate polymerisation.
- Composition of the material: composites with a high loading of small particles may tend to scatter more light than materials with a relatively low loading of larger particles and, as such, may have relatively limited depth of cure.
- The temperature of the material: composite materials warmed prior to curing exhibit superior physical properties (owing to increased polymerisation) compared with materials that are polymerised when cold. Furthermore, composites warmed in a composite heater may have superior flow characteristics to cold composites.

- The presence of oxygen: oxygen in the ambient atmosphere inhibits the polymerisation of the surface layer of composite resin materials. This can cause difficulties in placing an aesthetic restoration of an appropriate lustre but is advantageous when wishing successive increments of composite resin to bond to each other.

Finally, How Do We Do It?

The description below covers the placement of composite resin in an occlusal cavity, special placement techniques for the restoration of proximal and occlusoproximal cavities are described in Chapter 7. Finishing and polishing techniques are described in Chapter 8.

It is assumed that the cavity has already been prepared (Chapter 4) and that the pulp and dentine have been protected in an appropriate manner (Chapter 5), including application of a suitable adhesive system.

- Select a composite material of filler:resin ratio in excess of 60% by volume.

- It is useful when restoring posterior cavities with composite resin to select a shade of material which is slightly lighter than the surrounding tooth tissue. This facilitates discrimination between the restoration and natural tooth at the time of finishing, let alone when the restoration needs to be replaced or refurbished. The possible exception to this approach is when there is buccal exposure of a mesial box in a maxillary premolar. Otherwise, the slight mismatch in shade should in no way compromise the patient's dental attractiveness. Some commercially available composite materials include separate enamel and dentine shades. These should be considered for use in regions where an aesthetic appearance is critical.

- Composite resin materials are supplied in either syringes or compules (Figs 6-8 and 6-9). Syringed materials need to be placed on a parchment pad and applied to the cavity using a placement instrument, such as a flat plastic. Materials supplied in compules are best applied directly to the cavity, but they may be dispensed and applied in a similar fashion to syringed material. Best available evidence indicates that direct placement into the cavity using a compule gives the best clinical outcome in terms of adaptation and limiting the number of voids within both the body and the interfaces of restorations. Care should be taken to replace

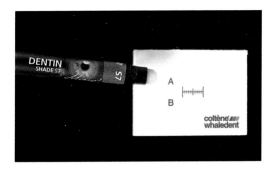

Fig 6-8 Composite material available in syringes.

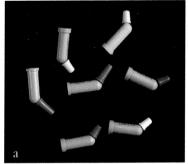

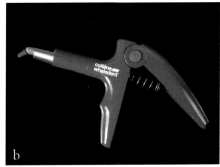

Fig 6-9 Composite material available in compules (sometimes referred to as "injectable"). (a) The compules. (b) The hand-held "gun" used for dispensing the composite.

the caps on syringes to prevent partial polymerisation of the remaining material by ambient or operatory light. Compules are intended for single-patient use and should not be reused in the interests of infection control. Some manufacturers produce "composite heaters". These devices allow preheating of syringes or compules in order to reduce the viscosity of the resin composite and thereby increase flowability and adaptation to cavities.

- Composite materials are generally sticky in nature. It is important to remember that adherence to the placement instrument can result in the material lifting or displacing during application; as a result, voids or marginal defects may be incorporated in the restoration. This can be avoided by using spreading rather than dabbing actions to apply the material, using good quality placement instruments (Fig 6-10) with polished rather than scratched surfaces, or even using Teflon-coated

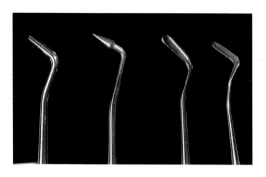

Fig 6-10 Specialised and good-quality composite placement instruments.

instruments, and, most importantly, limiting the working of the material in the cavity. Under no circumstances should the placement instrument be dipped in bonding agent, alcohol or water, let alone any other fluid, to prevent the material sticking to the instrument. Such techniques have adverse consequences on the physical properties of the newly placed restoration.

- Composite materials should be applied and adapted to cavities in increments not greater than 2 mm in thickness. Even smaller increments should be considered for materials that are dark in shade or when placing composite in deep portions of cavities that are inaccessible to the light-curing guide. Successive increments should not link opposing cusps or cavity walls but should instead be applied obliquely from one cavity wall to the base of the opposing cavity wall (see Fig 6-2).

- Increments of resin composite should be cured using either a QTH or LED light-curing unit. The activating light should be delivered as close to the material being cured as possible (Figs 6-11 and 6-12). As the light emitted from a light-curing light guide can be harmful to the naked eye, if looked at directly, a light shield should be used. The power output of QTH lights should be checked on a regular basis using a light meter. Curing times should be adhered to meticulously. No harm comes from more light than is regular, whereas shortening curing times can have significant detrimental effect.

- When applying the surface increment in the placement of a light-cured composite restoration, the material should be sculpted while soft,

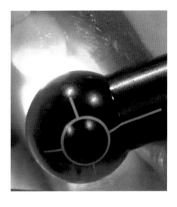

Fig 6-11 When curing the surface of the composite restoration, the light-curing guide should be placed as close to the surface as possible (this image shows composite being cured with a second-generation light-emitting diode curing light).

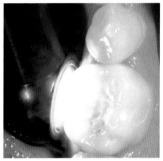

Fig 6-12 It is also useful when curing the composite restoration to direct the curing light from the buccal and lingual surfaces.

incorporating the required anatomy into the restoration. As oxygen inhibition of the surface increment can limit the ability to polish the restoration, the surface should be slightly over-built prior to curing. This facilitates "polishing back" of the surface layer to leave a well-cured surface, with best possible surface finish.

Key Learning Points

- Proper isolation is essential when placing successful posterior composite restorations; however, rubber dam use is not mandatory.
- Appropriate material selection is critical to the success of posterior composites.
- Light-activated composite resins are the "material of choice". Light-curing units of the QTH or LED type should be used.

- A composite resin restoration should not be placed in bulk or cured in bulk; it should be built up in increments in such a way as to minimise the effects of poymerisation contraction.
- Curing times must not be shortened, if anything they should be lengthened when curing deeply placed materials or ones of a dark shade.

Further Reading

Brunthaler A, Konig F, Lucas T, Sperr W, Schedle A. Longevity of direct resin composite restorations in posterior teeth. Clin Oral Invest 2003;7:63–70.

Ray NJ, Lynch CD, Burke FM, Hannigan A. Early surface hardness of a resin composite exposed to a pulse-delayed curing exposure: a comparison of a tungsten halogen and a plasma arc lamp, in vitro. Eur J Prosthodont Restor Dent 2005;13:177–181.

Ray NJ, Lynch CD, Burke FM, Hannigan A. Early surface microhardness of a resin composite: a comparison of a tungsten halogen and a LED curing lamp, in vitro. Eur J Prosthodont Restor Dent 2006;14:7–12.

Rueggeberg FA, Blalock JS, Callan RS. LED curing lights: what's new? Compend Contin Educ Dent 2005;26:586–589.

Chapter 7

Getting Back in Touch: Restoring Proximal Contours

Aim

The aim of this chapter is to consider the various techniques available for restoring the proximal contours of proximal and occlusoproximal composite resin restorations in posterior teeth.

Outcome

Having read this chapter the reader will:
- appreciate the advantages and disadvantages of the various matrix systems and wedging techniques available to aid the appropriate placement of posterior composites
- understand how to create appropriate proximal contours in posterior composite restorations.

Introduction

One of the principal challenges in placing two- and three-surface occlusoproximal posterior composites is to restore the proximal contours fully and with appropriate contact areas.

Failure to provide an adequate contact area will result in "food packing", which will cause pain and gingival inflammation, and ultimately lead to periodontal destruction and secondary caries. Creation of overhangs will preclude effective cleaning of the gingival margins – focal points for pathogenic bacteria capable of causing periodontal disease and secondary caries (Fig 7-1).

Problems

Specific problems relating to the placement of composite resins in proximal cavities in posterior teeth include:
- it is difficult to ensure that material is fully polymerised and that polymerisation contraction has not resulted in a marginal gap along the gingival margin when light-curing composite resin at the base of the proximal box

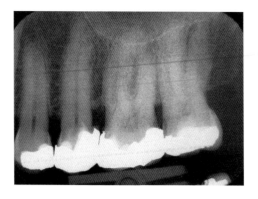

Fig 7-1 Intraoral radiograph including restored maxillary teeth with overhanging restorations. There is also evidence of interproximal bone loss.

- it is all too easy to fail to restore a tight, suitably contoured and located contact area
- it is difficult to contour and finish over-built composite restorations.

These difficulties can be largely addressed by careful selection of an appropriate matrix system and wedging technique. Great care must be taken to contour, place, adapt and wedge the selected matrix prior to commencing placement of the restoration. The sufficiency of the matrix and the wedging will not improve during the placement of the restoration.

Selecting a Matrix System and Wedge Technique

Matrices are, of themselves, of defined thickness, and the effect of this must be compensated for during placement. The use of an appropriate wedging technique is important in overcoming this difficulty. A wedge, in addition to adapting the matrix to the tooth to be restored, separates adjacent teeth. This separation allows the restoration to be built out to compensate for the thickness of the matrix. When the wedge is removed, the tooth returns to its original position and, if all goes according to plan, brings the adjacent teeth back into firm contact.

Matrix systems and wedges commonly described for the placement of posterior composites include:
- transparent matrix bands and light-transmitting wedges
- circumferential metal matrix bands and flexible/wooden wedges
- sectional metal matrices and flexible/wooden wedges.

Transparent matrix bands and light-transmitting wedges were introduced at a time when it was thought that composite resin materials contract on polymerisation in the direction of the polymerising light. Hence, if the tip of the light-curing guide was positioned over the occlusal surface of a cavity, as it would have to be if a metal matrix band were used, then it was thought that the composite resin material would shrink in an occlusal direction and, in the process, "lift" off the floor of the proximal box, creating a marginal gap. It is now known that this is not the case; composite resins do not shrink in the direction of the polymerising light but rather towards the portion of the cavity where the bond to tooth tissue is greatest, for example towards the thickest section of enamel. It is, therefore, a matter of some relief that transparent matrix bands can be dispensed with in procedures for the placement of posterior composites. The thickness, let alone the difficulties in handling and placing such bands, greatly complicates the placement procedure, with a substantial risk of compromising clinical outcomes with posterior composites.

In addition, light-curing wedges, notwithstanding doubts about their effectiveness, suffer the disadvantages of all rigid wedges. In particular, rigid wedges do not adapt the matrix band tightly along the curved proximal contour of the tooth. In contrast, they create a point contact between the matrix band and the tooth, increasing the likelihood of the formation of proximal overhangs (Fig 7-2).

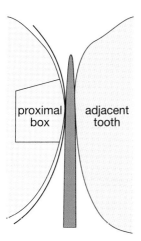

Fig 7-2 Use of a rigid wedge, such as a light-transmitting wedge, creates a point contact between the matrix and the curved cavosurface margin, increasing the likelihood of overhang formation.

Metal matrix systems used with a flexible wooden wedge offer many advantages over transparent matrices and light-transmitting wedges. When used in combination with an appropriate "layering" technique (Chapter 6), metal matrices with wooden wedges offer:

- a reduced risk of developing gaps between the composite restoration and the cavosurface margins of the cavity
- improved depth of cure, notably in the deeper region of the proximal box
- overall reduction in polymerisation contraction, which, amongst other advantages, is important in limiting residual stresses in the restored tooth unit.

Two groups of metal matrix systems are available:

- the traditional circumferential metal matrix system (e.g. Tofflemire and Siqveland systems; Fig 7-3)
- newer sectional metal matrices, which are adapted solely to the proximal region being restored (Fig 7-4).

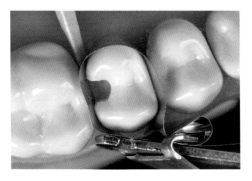

Fig 7-3 Example of a circumferential metal matrix system.

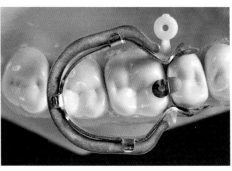

Fig 7-4 Example of a sectional metal matrix system (V-Ring, TrioDent Ltd, New Zealand).

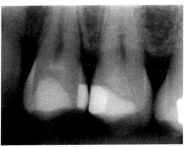

Fig 7-5 Restorations placed with a sectional and a circumferential metal band in the distal surface of the maxillary first premolar and the mesial surface of the maxillary second premolar, respectively. A curved contour was achieved using the sectional matrix; a flat contour had been previously achieved using the circumferential band.

Traditional circumferential metal matrix systems can be used to achieve a suitable clinical outcome. While such matrices can be contoured and burnished, they have been criticised on the grounds that they tend to produce a "flat" rather than contoured proximal surface (Fig 7-5).

Sectional metal matrices, in particular the recently introduced varieties, do not suffer such limitations. They may be held in place either with a wedge alone or with a sectional matrix retainer and a wedge. Many of the commercially available sectional metal matrices are thinner than the circumferential metal, let alone transparent, alternatives.

Most sectional metal matrices are precontoured. Such thin, preshaped matrix systems are capable of producing much better proximal contours than a relatively thick, metal matrix band, let alone a circumferential transparent matrix system.

Selection of an appropriate wedging technique is important when considering the dual aims of separating the teeth, to allow the contact area to be restored, and minimising the risk of proximal overhang formation. Flexible/wooden wedges of an appropriate size are indicated for this purpose (Fig 7-6).

It should be appreciated that as teeth separate and the wedge adapts to the contour of the tooth, the wedge typically needs to be pushed deeper into the interdental space, possibly on more than one occasion.

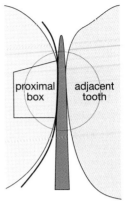

Fig 7-6 (left) Use of a flexible wedge, such as a wooden wedge, adapts the matrix to the curved cavosurface margin, thereby limiting the likelihood of overhang formation.

Contrast this to the use of a rigid wedge, such as a light-transmitting wedge (shown in Fig 7-2 and on the right here).

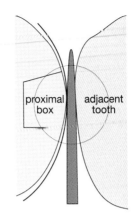

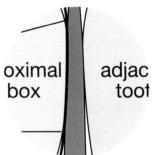

Enlarged views of the contact with the proximal box.

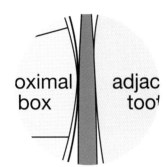

Creating a "Good" Contact

Following selection and application of the most appropriate matrix band and wedge, it is necessary to consider the most appropriate means of placing the composite resin material. Current evidence suggests that the best results are achieved by directly injecting composite into a preparation, and adapting the material, rather than attempting to pack or condense it. The less the composite is manipulated the better.

Techniques for creating a satisfactory proximal contact include:
- pressing a ball-ended or specially designed contact-forming instrument on to the adjacent tooth through the matrix while placing composite in the proximal region
- forming the "outer" proximal section of the restoration first, and then restoring the inner proximal and occlusal regions (Fig 7-7).

86

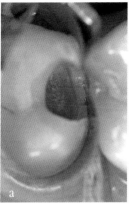 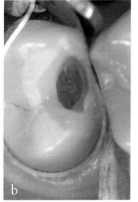 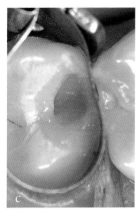

Fig 7-7 Restoration of a distal cavity (a) using composite resin. The missing proximal wall is first restored (b), followed by the internal portions using an oblique incremental technique (c).

This second technique offers the advantages of good visual access to the proximal region being restored, good moisture control when placing the restoration, particularly the "inner" regions of the restoration, and reduced risks of inadequate proximal contacts and formation of proximal overhangs. Other techniques that have been proposed for the placement of proximal composite restorations include placing an initial layer of flowable composite resin to line the floor of the proximal box. There is, at present, no evidence to suggest that this technique is associated with more favourable clinical outcomes than the currently advised direct application of composite resin using an incremental layering and curing technique.

In contrast, given the tendency of flowable composite resins to suffer void formation (as described in Chapter 2), their use may be found to be contraindicated. Other once popular techniques, such as the incorporation of glass–ionomer and prepolymerised composite inserts, have been discredited.

So All This Means ...

Proximal contacts created by means of either sectional or circumferential metal matrix bands and a flexible/wooden wedge are better than those created with transparent matrix bands and light-transmitting wedges.

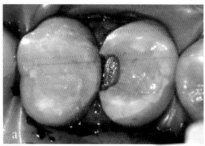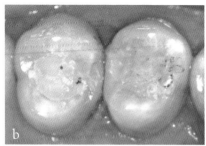

Fig 7-8 A distocclusal composite restoration had been placed in the maxillary first premolar and a mesiocclusal composite restoration in the maxillary second premolar; subsequently, the patient presented complaining of food packing. The contact was assessed and found to be deficient. (a) Composite was removed from the mesial surface of the maxillary second premolar. (b) A matrix system was applied, and fresh composite placed.

Based on current best-available evidence, the hierarchy of techniques available to restore proximal contours using composite resin is as follows:
1. Sectional metal matrix bands and flexible/wooden wedges (preferred)
2. Circumferential metal matrix bands and flexible/wooden wedges (clinically satisfactory results possible)
3. Transparent matrix bands and light-transmitting wedges (of limited value and to be avoided).

If the worst happens and a proximal contact is inadequate, let alone open, it is possible to correct the situation immediately by removing and replacing the deficient section of the restoration. As described in Chapter 9, the procedure, in a similar manner to a repair, involves removal of the proximal region of the newly placed composite restoration, selection and use of an appropriate bonding system, application of a suitable matrix and wedge, and rebuilding the contact area (Fig 7-8). Care should be taken to ensure that the new contact is satisfactory in terms of being tight, suitably located and well finished in order to limit interproximal wear in clinical service.

Boxing Clever: Ensuring that the Margin of the Proximal Box is Sealed

Placing composite resin in the base of the proximal box region can be fraught with difficulty. In this region:
- access for visual inspection and placement instruments may be compromised

- the remaining enamel, and hence the opportunity for a predictable bond, is limited
- moisture control is difficult.

Coupled with these problems, how are adequate irradiation and polymerisation achieved at the base of the proximal box?

There are a number of hints that are helpful in overcoming these specific problems.

- The proximal cavosurface margins, in particular those in the apical portion of the proximal box, should not be finished with bevels. Cavity preparation (Chapter 4) will create intra-enamel bevels best suited to achieving optimal bonding. What little enamel is present in the apical portion of a suitably prepared proximal box is to be conserved rather than further reduced.

- If the gingival margin of the proximal box is formed of dentine and cementum, and is located subgingivally, then it may be more appropriate to place a resin-modified glass–ionomer cement (RMGIC) base extending out the gingival margin prior to placing the composite resin restoration: the open-sandwich technique. The RMGICs are preferable to traditional glass–ionomer cements in this situation, as the traditional cements tend to "wash out" along the gingival margin: the most common site for secondary caries in all forms of occlusoproximal restorations. While the use of a RMGIC probably improves the quality of the marginal seal along a subgingivally located gingival margin of dentine and cementum, some evidence suggests that the use of open-sandwich techniques can reduce the fracture resistance of the restored tooth unit. If a gingival margin of dentine and cementum is located supragingivally and accessible for interproximal cleaning, then it should be possible to achieve gingival marginal seal by means of dentine bonding only.

- Avoid moisture contamination of the proximal box. If moisture occurs, as may be the case from time to time irrespective of the method selected for moisture isolation, it must not be ignored. Any contamination of the box, let alone the rest of the preparation will severely compromise adaptation, bonding and, in turn, seal. A contaminated preparation must be washed and dried prior to repeating bonding, including etching as indicated clinically as part of the bonding procedure.

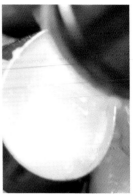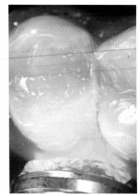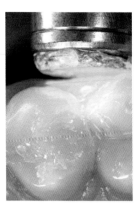

Fig 7-9 Irradiation of composite: (a) The surface increment of the composite material was irradiated from the occlusal surface. (b,c) Following removal of the matrix, the completed restoration was irradiated from the palatal and buccal surfaces.

- Apply the selected materials in strict accordance with manufacturer's directions for use.

- Following removal of the matrix band and wedge, the newly placed composite resin restoration should be "trans-irradiated" with curing light from both the buccal and lingual/palatal surfaces (Fig 7-9).

- Finish the margins of the restorations using atraumatic techniques.

Finally, How Do We Do It?

Following completion of cavity preparation and the protection of dentine and pulp, typically by means of the application of an adhesive bonding system, the following steps are taken.

1. Select and place a sectional metal matrix band supported and adapted with a flexible/wooden wedge, which should cause some separation of the teeth. When restoring three-surface occlusoproximal cavities, simultaneous mesial and distal wedging should be avoided as this tends to result in extrusion of the prepared tooth rather than the intended separation.

2. Burnish the matrix against the adjacent tooth to create a contact area of suitable size and shape.

3. Apply and adapt an approximately 1 mm thick increment of composite resin to the base of the proximal box. Composite resin is not "tooth-coloured amalgam". No attempt should be made to condense the material in the proximal box.

4. Use a layering technique to restore the apical portion of the box. Do not "link" the opposing proximal walls with a single increment.

5. Create the proximal surfaces of the restoration prior to restoring the occlusal portion. This facilitates the maintenance of moisture control and completion of the restoration.

6. Complete the restoration of the cavity. A layering technique should be used throughout the process, with increments not exceeding 2 mm in depth.

7. Following removal of the metal matrix, additionally irradiate the proximal box from both the buccal and lingual direction.

8. Ensure that no proximal overhangs have been created during placement. Should proximal overhangs be present, these must be removed using appropriate contouring and finishing instrumentation and techniques as described in Chapter 8.

9. Assess the quality of the proximal contact using dental floss. If the contact point is light, let alone open, consideration should be given to effecting an immediate adjustment, involving the removal and replacement of the contact area.

Key Learning Points

- Restoring the proximal contour and contact area is important to the initial sufficiency and subsequent clinical performance of occluso-proximal posterior composites.
- Composite resin materials suffer polymerisation contraction and, as a consequence, require incremental placement to avoid marginal gap formation, in particular along the gingival margin.
- Selection of an appropriate matrix and wedging system is crucial to restoring the proximal contour and contact. Current best evidence suggests that best results are achieved using a precontoured sectional metal matrix and flexible/wooden wedge.

- Should the contact area be insufficient, let alone open, it should be revised by removal of the contact area, placement of a new matrix and wedge and the build up of a new contact area.

Further Reading

Loomans BA, Opdam NJ, Roeters FJ, Bronkhorst EM, Burgersdijk RC, Dorfer CE. A randomized clinical trial on proximal contacts of posterior composites. J Dent 2006;34:292–297.

Mullejans R, Badawi MO, Raab WH, Lang H. An in vitro comparison of metal and transparent matrices used for bonded Class II resin composite restorations. Oper Dent 2003;28:122–126.

Chapter 8

Almost There: Finishing Techniques

Aim

The aim of this chapter is to consider the various instruments and techniques available for finishing posterior composite restorations.

Outcome

Having read this chapter, the reader will:
- be aware of various finishing instruments and techniques available for posterior composites
- appreciate the significance of appropriate finishing techniques in producing a satisfactory restoration and in minimising the risk of future disease and the need for further operative intervention.

Introduction

For many busy practitioners, the potential exists for regarding the finishing of composite restorations as an after-thought to the main event of placing the restoration. The most difficult part of the clinical procedure has been completed and there is a danger of thoughts drifting on to the next procedure or patient while "going through the motions" of finishing the newly placed restoration. Herein lies a risk to the longevity of the restoration: injudicious and careless finishing will damage the restoration, with the potential to cause early marginal deterioration, leakage, secondary caries and, if the adjacent soft tissues are traumatised, loss of gingival contour, recession and possibly the initiation of periodontal disease. Further consequences of injudicious and careless finishing may include excessive heat production, with damage to the limiting surface layer of composite, if not the pulp; iatrogenic damage to tooth surfaces adjacent to the restoration; damage to adjacent teeth; and loss of carefully restored occlusal and proximal contacts.

How Should Posterior Composite Restorations be Finished?

The aim of finishing posterior composite restorations is to refine the contour and contacts, optimise marginal adaptation and to give the restoration as smooth a surface as possible. Finishing will also enhance the aesthetic qualities of the restoration and facilitate cleaning as part of the patient's routine oral hygiene procedures. Finishing, including the identification of any deficiencies in the newly placed restoration, is greatly aided by the use of magnification in the form of loupes.

The Occlusal Surface

The occlusal surface of the restoration often includes "high spots" and may require generalised reduction if it has been over-built to avoid leaving the surface of restoration limited by an air-inhibited layer. Such a surface layer, if not removed in finishing, can be susceptible to staining and atypical wear of the completed restoration. Following removal of the rubber dam, articulating paper should be used to identify "high spots" and guide any necessary reduction and refinement of the occlusal contours. Occlusal contacts should be assessed in both maximum intercuspation and lateral excursive movements. If occlusal contacts are harmonious with the patient's existing occlusal scheme, then care should be taken not to inadvertently remove them in over-zealous polishing (Fig 8-1). Occlusal contacts occurring at the tooth–restoration interface are not welcome, as they can lead to early marginal failure (Fig 8-2). If the likelihood of such contact was not identified prior to cavity preparation and placement of the restoration, the only option available may be to adjust the contour of the opposing tooth. If such action is necessary, it is important to have the consent of the patient, who may well think that something is amiss. The adjustment to opposing tooth should shift rather than eliminate the contact giving cause for concern.

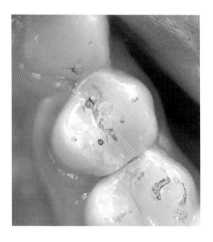

Fig 8-1 Occlusal contacts on a newly placed composite restoration. As occlusal contacts are observed on the adjacent teeth, the restoration is not causing any occlusal interference. There is no requirement to remove further composite from the occlusal surface of this restoration.

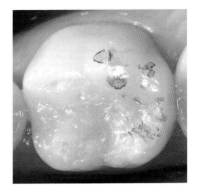

Fig 8-2 Occlusal contacts occurring at the distolingual tooth–restoration interface. This is undesirable; the opposing occlusal contact should be moved, not removed, to avoid marginal failure.

Instrumentation

Adjustment of the occlusal surface of the completed restoration is best achieved using rotary instrumentation. Coarse diamonds should not be used for this purpose as these tend to cause deep scratching, and some filler particle pluck-out in the surface of the restoration, let alone eliminate whatever contour has been incorporated in the restoration (Fig 8-3). These effects are minimised by the use of fine and superfine composite-finishing diamond burs and multi-fluted composite-finishing tungsten carbide burs. Whatever type of composite-finishing bur is used, care should be taken to limit iatrogenic damage to the tooth tissues adjacent to the restoration. To help to limit such damage, finishing burs should be used with light operating pressures, avoiding contact wherever possible with the adjacent tooth surfaces. This may be best achieved by always directing the bur on to the restoration rather than from the middle of the restoration towards the adjacent tooth surfaces, let alone across the margin in an attempt to enhance

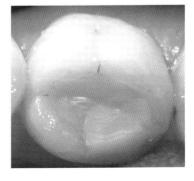

Fig 8-3 Composite restoration that has been finished inappropriately. The parallel scratch marks on the restoration surface were most likely caused by a coarse rotary finishing bur.

adaptation. Restorations should not be "over-carved" to reproduce deep fissure systems and other occlusal features. Apart from making the restoration more difficult to clean, deep fissures and related features can predispose the restoration to fracture. The aim of contouring is to create a somewhat rounded form of the original morphology of the tooth.

Finishing burs are available in a variety of sizes and shapes. A range of finishing burs is required for effective contouring of composite restorations of different sizes and outline in premolar and molar teeth.

Water Cooling
Heat generation during finishing can damage the surface of the restoration, traumatise underlying dentine and possibly cause pulpal damage. In addition to applying finishing instruments intermittently and with light operating pressures to limit heat generation, copious water cooling should be used in conjunction with all rotary instruments. Effective water cooling greatly reduces the adverse effects of heat generation, with the advantage of washing away debris, improving vision and limiting undesirable three-body wear caused by debris being retained between the finishing instrument and the surface being finished.

Magnification
The use of magnification, such as loupes, greatly enhances the quality of the finishing of restorations, both in terms of surface finish and the quality of the margins. Given the dimension to which one must work to achieve good clinical outcomes, the use of magnification aids, notably loupes, should be routine (Fig 8-4).

Finishing Tasks
Following contouring of the restoration, further refinements and polishing can be completed using a range of instruments and devices, including graded series of finishing discs, composite-finishing and polishing points and polishing pastes applied using polishing cups. The selection and use of these instruments and devices is determined by the morphology and, to a lesser extent, the size and location of the restoration. As in all operative procedures, finishing instruments and devices must be used in strict accordance with the manufacturer's directions for use, including typically the need to work intermittently with light operating pressures and, where appropriate, water cooling. To achieve a good surface finish, irregularities in the surface of the restoration must be progressively reduced in size using progressively finer instruments and abrasives. At each stage, the irregularities in the surface being finished should be as uniform as possible.

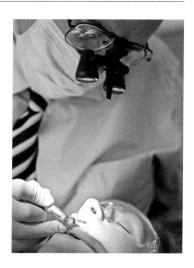

Fig 8-4 The use of magnification is advised during finishing procedures.

The margins of the completed restoration should be assessed visually using magnification and tactilely using an explorer. Any deficiencies should be identified and managed appropriately, possibly by means of a localised repair. The use of a bonding agent to "seal" the surface and margins of a completed posterior composite restoration is considered good practice, even if visible marginal defects are not present. Small microscopic defects may be present and the use of a bonding agent, if suitably applied, may prevent these defects enlarging or in some other way compromising the restoration. The application of a bonding agent to a newly finished composite restoration will increase its lustre, thereby improving appearance and the feeling of "smoothness" for the patient (Fig 8-5). The patient should, however, be warned that the surface of restorations treated in this way may feel a little sticky for a few hours, until such time as the air-inhibited limiting layer has been lost.

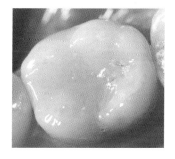

Fig 8-5 Completed occlusal composite restoration in a mandibular first molar. (Restoration made in Miris 2, Coltène Whaledent, Switzerland).

Just When You Thought It Was All Over:
Finishing Proximal Surfaces

Finishing proximal surfaces of posterior composite restorations presents special difficulties. Access is limited to assess the quality of the surface, detect localised defects and for the use of conventional finishing instruments. Notwithstanding limited access, it is critical that any undesirable surface features and defects are managed. In addition, the presence of overhanging margins can lead to the development of secondary caries and periodontal disease and, as a consequence, cannot be ignored.

Following removal of any wedges, matrix system and, if used, the rubber dam, proximal surfaces must be inspected and assessed most carefully. Initially, this may be achieved visually, with special emphasis on good light conditions and the use of magnification. Thereafter, it is useful to assess the restoration surface and the tooth–restoration interface by lightly drawing a dental explorer across the surfaces of the restored tooth to detect the presence of marginal excesses, overhangs and defects. It is also important that the adequacy of the proximal contact is assessed using dental floss (Chapter 7), which may also be used to detect gingival overhangs.

Rotary instruments may be used to finish accessible margins of proximal restorations, but only with great care to avoid damage to adjacent teeth. Composite finishing strips, which may include a section of relatively coarse abrasive for contouring, can be effective at removing thin-section marginal excesses, but they may not be very effective at reducing gingival overhangs of some substance. When using finishing strips, it is important to avoid inadvertently removing the proximal contact and flattening the proximal contour. To remove gingival overhangs, and otherwise contour the apical portion of proximal posterior composites, consideration should be given to using specially designed sonic tips or safe-sided, fine-grit, diamond-coated contouring and finishing tips for use in specially designed reciprocating handpieces.

While such devices can be very effective, care must be exercised not to damage tooth surfaces adjacent to the restoration irreversibly, in particular the root surface apical to the gingival margin of the restoration. Such damage runs the risk of the patient suffering persistent post-operative sensitivity, which could necessitate further operative intervention. The best treatment for proximal overhangs is prevention, through careful selection and use of the most appropriate matrix and wedge system.

The presence of marginal voids in proximal sections of posterior composites presents special diagnostic and management difficulties. Marginal voids that are visible and accessible may be managed in the same manner as those occurring on occlusal surfaces, as described above. If, however, marginal voids are present in inaccessible areas, notably the central portion of the gingival margin (the most common site for secondary caries), then consideration should be given to repeating the placement of the restoration. This will be in the best interest of the patient as attempts to effect repairs in such situations typically go from bad to worse.

The ideal approach for marginal voids is prevention, similar to the avoidance of overhangs. It is much better to spend time meticulously following recommended procedures for the placement of posterior composites than attempting to make good a restoration with defects and deficiencies: the latter inevitably involves compromises, let alone considerable frustration.

The final challenge when finishing occlusoproximal composite restorations is the creation of a satisfactory marginal ridge and occlusal embrasure space. The marginal ridge region is best contoured with fine diamond, or multi-fluted tungsten carbide finishing burs. The height of the marginal ridge in the new restoration should match that of the marginal ridge in the adjacent tooth, occlusal clearance permitting. Particular attention needs to be paid to the proximal face of the marginal ridge and to the restoration of the sluice ways, buccally and lingually. These features are important in limiting the risk of proximal food packing, even in the presence of a satisfactory contact area.

In summary, it is important to realise that the finishing of posterior composite restorations has a significant part to play in the success of the restoration and the in-service performance of the restored tooth unit. Chair-side time spent in the effective finishing of composite restorations is time well spent.

Key Learning Points

- The finishing of posterior composite restorations is very important to the survival of the restoration.
- Use of appropriate finishing techniques can limit the risk of future disease recurrence and progression and minimise the need for future operative intervention.
- When finishing composite restorations, a key consideration is minimising iatrogenic damage to the restoration, the remaining tooth tissues and adjacent teeth.

Chapter 9
The Management of Failing Direct Composite Restorations: Replace or Repair?
Igor R Blum

Aim

Managing a composite restoration with localised defects is a common clinical situation. The repair of such a restoration is a minimally interventive means of extending the longevity of the restoration without unnecessarily sacrificing healthy tooth structure. This chapter aims to provide an overview of current knowledge and understanding of restoration repair in the clinical management of defective composite restorations. Additionally, some information is presented on the repair of tooth fracture adjacent to restorations.

Outcome

This chapter is intended to give insight into the indications, importance and benefits of restoration repair, together with details of relevant operative techniques aimed at conserving as much sound tooth structure as possible.

Introduction

Composite restorations, in common with all restorations, suffer deterioration and degradation in clinical service. The management of composite restorations with localised defects is, therefore, a common challenge in clinical practice. A "drill-and-fill" approach to the management of defective composite restorations that exhibit minor imperfections, which involves total removal of the defective restoration, is based on a flawed mechanistic rather than scientific style of operative dentistry. The result is the removal of the entire restoration and progressive cavity enlargement, with the unnecessary removal of sound tooth tissue. This leads to an acceleration of the downward spiral of a restored tooth, with its associated detrimental consequences: weakening of the tooth; repeated insults to the pulp, with increased risk of pulp death (Fig 9-1); and a misuse of patients' time, resources and tolerance to accept interventive dental care.

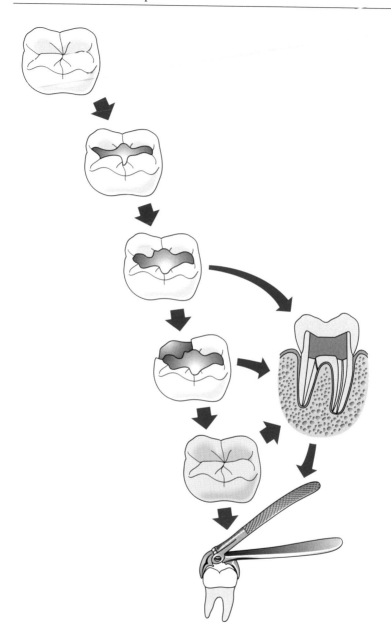

Fig 9-1 The downward spiral of a restored tooth.

It has been suggested that dental practitioners spend much of their chair-side time on the management of failing restorations. The reasons most commonly cited for replacing a direct composite restoration include:

- secondary caries as diagnosed clinically
- marginal defects
- marginal discoloration and staining
- incorrect shade of the restoration
- bulk discoloration
- bulk fracture of the restoration
- fracture of adjacent tooth issue
- wear of the restoration.

While some restorations will inevitably require replacement, it is suggested that many deteriorating, yet serviceable, restorations may be given extended longevity through repair procedures. It is clearly preferable, therefore, to perform a composite repair (i.e. partial replacement of the composite restoration, allowing preservation of that portion of the composite restoration which presents no clinical or radiographic evidence of failure) as an alternative to restoration replacement wherever possible. The repair of a composite restoration may include an element of refurbishment, a procedure that should normally pre-empt and delay repair, let alone replacement. Refurbishment procedures typically involve the refinishing or resurfacing of a restoration, with or without recontouring. Refinishing may be limited to the margins of a restoration and resurfacing may involve all of the exposed restoration surfaces.

Advantages of Repair

The advantages of repairing localised defects in composite restorations include:

- preservation of tooth structure
- increased longevity of the restoration
- reduction of potentially harmful effects on the dental pulp
- reduction in treatment time
- reduced costs to the patient
- good patient acceptance
- no need for local anaesthesia, provided the repair is not extensive.

Criteria for Repair

Many factors play a role in the selection of repair over replacement of direct composite restorations with localised defects. These include the patient's risk status for caries, the clinical condition of the restored tooth unit and the cost/benefit assessments. Criteria for repair as opposed to complete restoration replacement can be broadly divided into two categories: patient-centred and tooth-specific criteria.

Patient-centred Criteria

Dentally motivated and informed patients who attend on a regular basis, maintain a good standard of oral health, and in whom the restorations can be monitored regularly are good candidates for composite repair procedures. Another group of suitable candidates for repair procedures are those who have complex medical histories or limited capacity to cooperate. In such patients, the nature of the intervention should be limited in terms of time and complexity. Refurbishment procedures can often be accomplished without the need for local anaesthesia and are, therefore, especially advantageous for patients with complex medical histories.

It is important that patients understand the nature of the repair procedure and how this procedure differs from restoration replacement. In obtaining informed consent for a composite repair procedure, it is essential to outline the disadvantages of the replacement strategy in terms of its effect on the longevity of the restored tooth unit. Similarly, the advantages of the repair strategy in terms of preserving tooth structure and its minimally inter-ventional nature must be explained.

In deciding whether to repair or replace a composite restoration in the presence of secondary caries, the decision to repair rather than replace is more likely to be correct in a patient with a low risk of further disease. If the decision is made to replace, rather than repair the restoration in such a low-risk patient, the preparation will be enlarged unnecessarily and the tooth inappropriately weakened. The longevity of the replacement restoration may be uncertain and it may carry increased risk of more complex and costly subsequent treatment, including endodontic therapy. Notwithstanding these short-comings, the replacement restoration may be subjected to the same, possibly unrecognised, limitations of the original restoration.

Tooth-specific Criteria

Having ascertained that patient-centred criteria are satisfied, tooth-specific criteria must be considered. To assess tooth-specific criteria, it is important to employ an appropriate selection of investigative techniques, no one investigative technique being sufficient to provide all the necessary information. Magnification aides for visual inspection and the interpretation of radiographic images are considered invaluable in maximising the sensitivity and specificity of clinical assessments.

Clinical Indications for Restoration Repair

Secondary Caries

Caries adjacent to the margin of a composite restoration (secondary caries) should be treated as a new primary lesion. As with all patients who present with a new lesion, preventive measures should be initiated, followed by operative intervention as and when the lesion is shown to be active and progressing through dentine, or cavitation has occurred. Operative intervention should be minimally interventive coupled with partial replacement of that portion of the adjacent composite restoration that has been undermined by the caries or that hinders the access required for effective caries removal. The portion of the composite restoration that presents no clinical or radiographic evidence of failure should be left in place, unless there is good clinical indication to resort to total restoration replacement with its various consequences.

Marginal Defects and Marginal Staining

It is important to realise that the presence of marginal defects does not always indicate the presence of secondary caries. If limited, marginal defects can be simply managed using refinishing procedures. Minor marginal defects in the occlusal surfaces of posterior composite restorations that are imperceptible to the patient are best monitored, with intervention being delayed until there is evidence of plaque accumulation, food stagnation or discoloration, which may herald progressive deterioration. Marginal defects in anterior composite restorations are more problematic because of their tendency to pick up exogenous stain. Refinishing coupled, where necessary, with refurbishment of the restoration is typically the most effective way to manage such staining successfully (Fig 9-2). If heavy, penetrating staining is present, total restoration replacement may be required to obtain a high-quality aesthetic outcome.

Superficial Colour Correction

If an incorrect shade had been selected for a previously placed composite restoration, this may be managed by resurfacing using a different shade of composite material. Wherever possible, the same restorative material should be used as the composite substrate, but this might not be possible if the restoration was placed by a different practitioner, details of the material used were not recorded in the patient's notes, or the previously placed material is no longer commercially available.

105

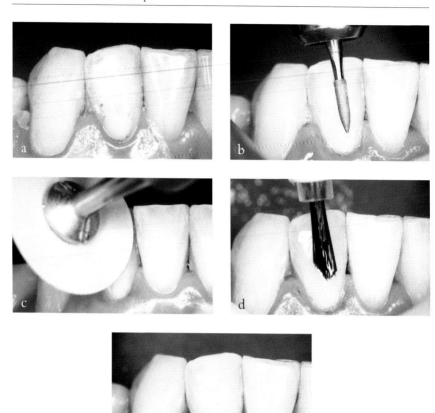

Fig 9-2 Treatment of staining: (a) Staining associated with otherwise satisfactory composite in the right mandibular lateral incisor. (b) Fine-particle diamond finishing bur used to remove stain and smooth the composite surface. (c) Flexible disk used to polish the composite surface. (d) Application of unfilled resin as a surface glaze (e) Refinished restoration after light curing of resin applied to the surface. (From Wilson, Roulet, Fuzzi, *Advances in Operative Dentistry*, Vol 2. London: Quintessence, 2001.)

Bulk Fracture

When a patient presents with a bulk fracture of a composite restoration, in particular soon after restoration placement, it is important to diagnose and eliminate the reason for the fracture, for example excess occlusal loading. This is necessary to avoid recurring bulk fracture, let alone a fracture including remaining tooth tissue. Bulk fracture of a composite restoration that has been in clinical service for many years is likely to be the result of stress fatigue within the composite material. If the bulk fracture is limited (less than half of the restoration), repair may be indicated; however, the integrity of the remaining portion of the restoration should be carefully assessed (Fig 9-3).

Fracture of Adjacent Tooth Tissue
Fracture of tooth tissue adjacent to a composite restoration may occur for various reasons, including parafunctional activity, trauma or subsequent to damaging polymerisation stresses at the time of restoration placement. A repair may be indicated if the cause of the fracture can be accurately diagnosed and, as a consequence, the risk of further fracture minimised, possibly through a preventive measure such as the provision of a mouthguard for a bruxist patient.

Wear of the Restoration
As wear of a composite restoration may have been accompanied by passive eruption, or at least tilting of the opposing tooth or teeth, the situation needs to be assessed most carefully. If the wear of the restoration is of a limited nature, confined to the occlusal surface and space exists to effect a repair,

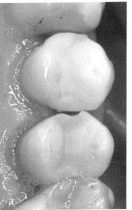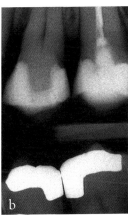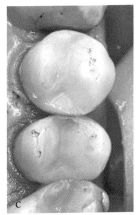

Fig 9-3 A 10-year-old posterior composite with a limited fracture of the marginal ridge and a cervical radiolucency indicative of secondary caries. (a) Clinical appearance. (b) Radiographic appearance. (c) Restoration following repair, including extension to manage the cervical secondary caries diagnosed radiographically. (Courtesy of N H F Wilson, *Minimally Invasive Dentistry*. London: Quintessence, 2007.)

then the situation may be resolved by resurfacing the restoration. If the wear involves a proximal surface and no space exists to restore the anatomic form of the restoration, then an alternative restorative approach may be indicated.

Contraindications for Repair

Contraindications for repair include:

- patient reluctance to accept a repair as an alternative to restoration replacement
- irregular attenders
- patients with a high risk of caries
- presence of caries undermining most of the composite restoration
- history of failure of a previous repair.

Clinical Procedure

The clinical procedure for the repair of a failing direct composite restoration is as follows.

1. Use local analgesia, as indicated clinically.

2. Remove the defective part of the composite restoration and any adjacent secondary caries.

3. Ensure adequate moisture control as it is essential to protect the preparation from contamination. This is best achieved with a rubber dam or judicious use of cotton wool rolls and salivary ejectors.

4. Protect the pulp according to current regimens.

5. The composite substrate is then roughened using either an intraoral sandblaster (CoJet-Sand, 3M ESPE, Germany; Microetcher, Danville Engineering Company, USA) or a diamond bur. Any exposed tooth tissue should also be roughened by sandblasting or with a bur to ensure the removal of any residual composite or pellicle in order to provide a fresh surface for bonding. The CoJet sandblaster utilises silica sand particles with a mean particle size of 30 μm. Research findings suggest that this provides a microretentive roughened and silicatised surface that enhances the strengths of the repair composite

binding to the composite substrate. If the composite substrate has not been treated by sandblasting, it must be acid etched together with the preparation margins for 15–30 seconds and then gently washed and dried using a three-in-one syringe. In addition to producing a favourable substrate surface for bonding, acid etching has a favourable cleansing effect.

6. The substrate surface then needs to be primed. If the composite substrate has been treated with the CoJet sandblaster, a silane primer and corresponding adhesive (e.g. ESPE Sil and Visio-Bond, 3M ESPE) is applied to the substrate and an adhesive bonding system to the adjacent tooth tissues and preparation margins, according to the manufacturer's directions. If the substrate has been acid etched, an adhesive bonding system should be applied to the acid-etched composite substrate and adjacent tooth tissues and preparation margins, according to the manufacturer's directions.

   Alternatively, a commercially available composite repair system (e.g. Ecusit-Composite Repair, DMG, Germany; Clearfil Repair Kit, Kuraray, Japan), which includes its own specifically formulated adhesive agent, may be used. While higher bond strengths have been reported in the literature using the CoJet system compared with traditional bonding procedures, only limited data exist, to date, about the difference in effectiveness between conventional adhesive systems and composite repair systems.

7. The resin-based composite material is then applied using a 2 mm incremental technique to repair the defect. Each increment must be polymerised using a visible light-curing unit. Ideally, the same type and brand of composite material should be used as the composite substrate, provided this information is known to the practitioner. The composite substrate must be at least 2 mm thick for the repair procedure to be successful.

8. The repair is then carefully contoured and finished using the current composite-finishing systems. The repair should be integrated imperceptibly into the restored tooth unit.

9. The occlusion should be checked and occlusal interferences, if present, corrected.

Repair of Fractured Tooth Tissue Adjacent to an Existing Amalgam Restoration

A further use of composite resin as a material of choice for restoration repair is in the repair of fractured tooth tissue adjacent to an existing amalgam restoration. Results from cross-sectional studies indicate that tooth fractures at such a location are a common occurrence. In particular, complete cusp fractures of posterior teeth have been reported to be commonly associated with amalgam restorations, with an incidence rate ranging between 4.4 and 14% over a two-year period.

As cuspal fractures are typically supragingival and a repair is more cost-effective and less invasive than restoration replacement, a repair should be considered wherever appropriate.

Despite a significant increase in intraoral repair systems available and a growing number of systems being introduced, let alone improvements in the techniques that facilitate alloy–resin bonding, there are few data on the longevity of bonded composite resin to amalgam surfaces in clinical service. In addition, there seems to be no consensus in the literature regarding the best method for repairing amalgam restorations with composite resin. The techniques most commonly described involve both (micro) mechanical retention and chemical adhesion, as outlined below.

Clinical Procedure

1. Use local analgesia, as indicated clinically.

2. Remove any undermined, unsupported tooth tissue and the surface of the amalgam restoration adjacent to the fracture to provide a fresh surface as a potential bonding substrate.

3. Prepare retention features within the amalgam restoration to provide mechanical retention for the composite material.

4. Ensure adequate moisture control as it is essential to protect the preparation from contamination. This is best achieved with a rubber dam or judicious use of cotton wool rolls and salivary ejectors.

5. The adjacent amalgam and tooth tissue surfaces are then roughened using either an intraoral aluminium oxide sandblaster (Microetcher, Danville Engineering Company, USA) or a diamond bur.

6. If indicated, provide any necessary pulp protection according to current regimens.

7. The tooth tissue surfaces are then acid etched for 15–30 seconds and thoroughly washed and dried using a three-in-one syringe.

8. The adhesive bonding system is applied to the conditioned tooth surfaces according to the manufacturer's directions.

9. An alloy-resin bonding agent (e.g. Alloy Primer, Kuraray, Japan) is applied to the roughened amalgam surface according to the manufacturer's directions.

10. A visible light-cure resin opaquer (e.g. Visiogem, 3M ESPE) is then applied to the conditioned amalgam surface. The opaquer has a similar chemistry as dental composite resin, and it chemically bonds to the alloy–resin bonding agent and composite resin.

11. The repair composite is placed using an incremental technique; each increment is fully light cured prior to applying a subsequent layer of material.

12. The repair is carefully contained and finished, with particular attention to ensuring that burs and finishing devices work from composite to the amalgam.

13. The occlusion should be checked and occlusal interferences, if present, corrected.

In clinical situations where an amalgam fracture has occurred, factors such as the existence of intact enamel/dentine, repair resins with different elastic moduli, surface chemical composition, morphology and age of the amalgam could also affect the adhesion of resin composites to amalgam surfaces.

Typical Bond Strength Values: How Well Will It Stick?

The typical bond strengths between composite resin and conditioned substrate surfaces are summarised in Table 9-1. These data should be borne in mind when considering and planning a repair procedure, in particular when the repaired tooth unit will be under heavy occlusal loading.

Table 9-1 **Shear bond strengths of composite resin (adherand) to various conditioned substrates**

Substrate	Adhesive	Shear bond strength (MPa)
Enamel	Conventional adhesive bonding systems	21–35
Dentine	Dentine adhesives	14–26
Aged composite	CoJet system	16–30
	Conventional adhesive bonding systems	12–20
Amalgam	Alloy bonding agents	3–6

Conclusion

The repair of failing composite restorations increases the longevity of the restorations. Repairs can provide excellent functional and aesthetic results while preserving that portion of the original composite restoration which remains serviceable. The use of an evidence-based repair protocol and up-to-date materials ensure the best clinical outcomes in the provision of repairs.

Given the lack of long-term randomised controlled clinical studies on the longevity of repaired restorations, it is important to monitor all such repairs on a regular basis.

Key Learning Points

- Many serviceable composite restorations can, over time, exhibit deterioration and degradation.
- It is recommended, in selected clinical situations, to repair or refurbish a deteriorating composite restoration rather than remove it in its entirety.
- New technologies, such as the use of intraoral sandblasters, have much to recommend them for use in such procedures.

Recommended Reading

Blum IR, Schriever A, Heidemann D, Mjör IA, Wilson, NHF. The repair of direct composite restorations: an international survey of the teaching of operative techniques and materials. Eur J Dent Educ 2003;7:41–48.

Hannig C, Laubach S, Hahn P, Attin T. Shear bond strength of repaired adhesive filling materials using different repair procedures. J Adhes Dent 2006;8:35–40.

Wilson, NHF, Setcos JC, Brunton PA. Replacement or repair of dental restorations. In Wilson NHF, Roulet J-F, Fuzzi M (eds.), Advances in Operative Dentistry, Vol.2: Challenges for the Future. Chicago, IL: Quintessence, 2001.

Chapter 10

Expanding Horizons: Advanced Uses of Posterior Composites

Aim

The aim of this chapter is to describe the placement of posterior composites in certain extended clinical situations.

Outcome

On completion of this chapter, the reader will be familiar with the placement of posterior composite restorations when:
• managing worn posterior teeth
• managing cracked tooth syndrome
• restoring endodontically treated teeth.

Introduction

Recent developments in the field of composite resin materials and associated bonding technologies, coupled with an increased understanding of relevant placement and handling techniques, have improved the success rates for posterior composites. With these improvements, applications of composite resin materials have expanded, with their use in the restoration of posterior teeth being no exception to the trend.

This chapter will consider three specific extensions of the use of composite resins in the restoration of posterior teeth: the management of worn teeth, dealing with cracked tooth syndrome and the restoration of the endodontically treated tooth. More extensive texts will have details of other uses, for example to change the shape of posterior teeth to facilitate the provision of removable partial dentures.

Managing Worn Posterior Teeth

Tooth surface loss is an increasingly common clinical phenomenon (Fig 10-1). As the term suggests, this condition involves the loss of tooth tissue from the surface of the affected tooth. Such loss can be attributed to three processes:

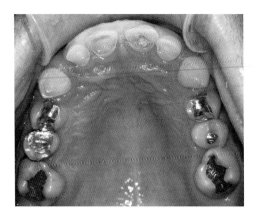

Fig 10-1 Unchecked tooth surface loss, in this case erosion, has caused loss of anterior tooth substance, with involvement of the pulp of the maxillary left central incisor.

- **attrition**: the loss by wear of tooth substance or a restoration caused by mastication or contact between occluding or proximal surfaces (Fig 10-2).
- **erosion**: the progressive loss of hard dental tissues by a chemical process not involving bacterial action (Figs 10-3 and 10-4).
- **abrasion**: the loss by wear of tooth substance or a restoration caused by factors other than tooth contact (Figs 10-5 and 10-6).

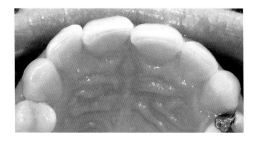

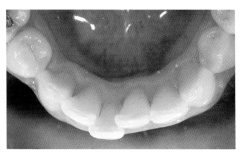

Fig 10-2 Mild attritional tooth surface loss affecting the maxillary and mandibular anterior teeth. Operative intervention may not be indicated at this stage; however provision of a nightguard and arrangements to monitor the wear with serial study casts is indicated.

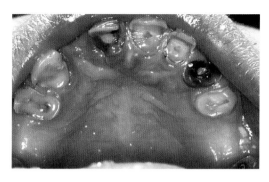

Fig 10-3 Advanced erosive tooth surface loss of maxillary anterior and posterior teeth in a 70-year-old former alcoholic.

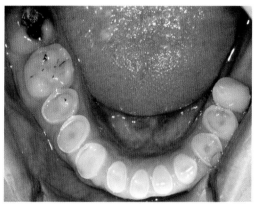

Fig 10-4 Advanced erosive tooth surface loss of mandibular anterior and posterior teeth in a 40-year-old former bulimic patient.

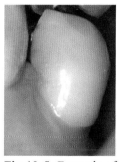

Fig 10-5 Example of abrasional tooth surface loss caused by overvigorous use of a toothbrush.

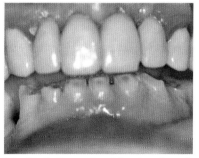

Fig 10-6 Example of abrasional tooth surface loss affecting the mandibular anterior teeth, caused by functional contact with unglazed porcelain on the palatal surface of the maxillary fixed bridge. (Courtesy of *Dental Update*).

117

Following occlusal tooth surface loss, it is common for axial tooth movement to occur. This movement, sometimes termed over- or supra-eruption, can pose challenges when restoring the affected tooth. Restoring worn posterior teeth can be difficult, possibly involving surgical crown lengthening and the placement of full-coverage crowns. This approach is, however, complicated, notwithstanding its aggressive nature and expense, let alone the risk of subsequent morbidity. An alternative treatment option is to consider the use of direct posterior composite restorations to restore the affected teeth.

As with any patient who presents with clinical signs and symptoms of tooth surface loss, it is important first to diagnose and manage the underlying cause of the problem. For example:
- attrition linked to bruxism: the patient should be managed, at least initially, using biteguard therapy (see Fig 10-2)
- erosion associated with excessive dietary acid intake: the patient should be given dietary counselling and monitored prior to planning any interventive dentistry (Fig 10-7)
- erosion from exposure to intrinsic acid: it is often best to liaise with the patient's general medical practitioner to arrange a referral to a gastroenterologist (see Fig 10-4)

It is also useful to use serial photographs and study casts to assess the rate and pattern of wear.

The approach to managing worn posterior teeth can broadly be divided into:
- relatively simple restoration of one or some affected teeth, where there has been little if any axial tooth movement
- complex restorations where many teeth have been affected, and axial tooth movement has occurred (Fig 10-8).

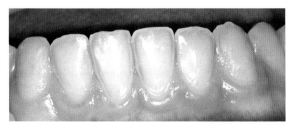

Fig 10-7 An example of erosive tooth surface loss caused by dietary intake. The patient had a habit of holding pieces of citrus fruit inside her lower lip; this resulted in tooth surface loss on the labial surfaces of the mandibular central incisor teeth.

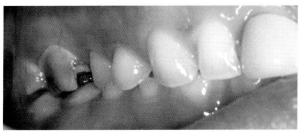

Fig 10-8 Following unchecked erosion of these posterior teeth, axial tooth movement has occurred. The management of this patient will not be straightforward.

The restoration of one or some affected teeth that have not undergone any axial tooth movement is often no more challenging than placing a direct intracoronal posterior composite, assuming there is space for the restoration and moisture isolation can be secured. More often than not, the most difficult aspect of the procedure is dealing with flat, tight, worn proximal contacts. The use of rubber dam is generally contraindicated as the occlusion must be checked as the restoration is built up incrementally. In the absence of axial movement subsequent to wear, the occlusion is generally managed using a conformative approach.

Management of complex posterior tooth wear is more challenging. It is possible, however, to achieve favourable clinical outcomes using composite resins. This approach is especially useful when wishing to provide transitional restorations to allow further monitoring of the dentition and the patient's ability to tolerate, in particular, an increase in vertical face height. According to the success of the composite restorations and the wishes of the patient, the transitional restorations can be monitored and maintained in anticipation of several years of clinical service, or they may be the prelude to further reconstructive treatment involving various forms of indirect restorations.

The following approach outlines the principles of one clinical approach to this situation (Fig 10-9).

Clinical Procedure

1. Once satisfied that the underlying cause of the tooth wear has been controlled, study casts of the worn dentition should be mounted in retruded contact position in a semiadjustable articulator.

119

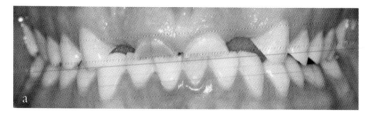

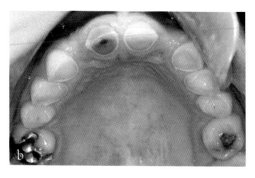

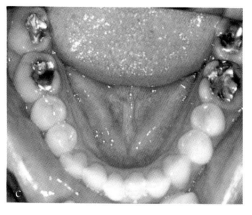

Fig 10-9 (a–c) A 30-year-old female patient who suffered from bulimia in the past. The patient has lost her maxillary lateral incisors, and has worn anterior and posterior teeth. There has been axial tooth movement, with over-eruption of the anterior and posterior teeth.

2. Subsequent to any necessary increase in vertical face height, a diagnostic wax-up of the planned alternations to the reorganised dentition should then be completed, together with a transparent blow-down matrix.

3. If not already attended to, the anterior teeth should be restored or modified to provide, where appropriate, canine or possibly anterior guidance.

4. Working according to a predetermined sequence, the posterior teeth are built up in twos or possibly groups of three, subsequent to any necessary preparation to round-off potential stress points and provide clear finishing lines.

5. Subsequent to etching and bonding in strict accordance with the manufacturer's directions, the composite resin material is applied with the aid of the matrix, thereby recreating the occlusal scheme developed in the diagnostic wax-up. If the build up of the occlusal surface requires a thickness of composite in excess of 2 mm, initial increments of composite should be applied and light cured prior to the use of the blow-down matrix (Fig 10-10).

Difficulty may be encountered when restoring adjacent teeth with the aid of a blow-down matrix, specifically in ensuring that teeth are not left bonded together at the level of the marginal ridge. Such difficulties may be avoided either by restoring alternate teeth or by restoring affected teeth individually and applying a separating medium to the adjacent teeth. Alternatively, an

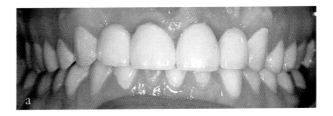

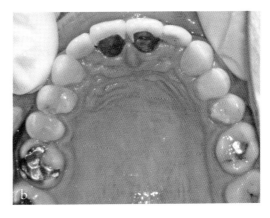

Fig 10-10 Management of the wear shown in Fig 10-9. (a) The worn posterior teeth were restored with composite resin. (b) The maxillary anterior teeth were restored using fixed bridgework.

appropriate matrix band and wedging system may be used for the initial restoration of the marginal ridge areas, but this has to be done in a way that will still allow the use of the blow-down matrix. While initial light curing may be achieved through the transparent blow-down matrix, further light curing will be required subsequent to its removal.

Following placement, the restorations must be carefully refined to eliminate any damaging interferences and ensure appropriate occlusal contacts. Time is required to finish the restorations satisfactorily and to ensure that the patient will be able to practise a high level of oral hygiene. Following such treatment, arrangements should be made to review the patient within a week to 10 days and thereafter as indicated clinically.

The use of direct composite restorations to restore worn posterior teeth has been criticised on the grounds that the restorations may have a limited lifespan compared with alternative treatment options, including gold castings, all-ceramic restorations and crowns. While it is acknowledged that directly placed posterior composites do not have the longevity of the alternative forms of restorations, the placement of extensive indirect restorations is an irreversible form of treatment, with an increased risk of tooth morbidity. The placement of composite resin restorations is, by contrast, minimally interventional, with more extensive forms of treatment always remaining an option. With further advances in the field of composite resin materials and associated bonding technologies, the applications of composites in the management of the worn dentition will increase.

Cracked Tooth Syndrome

Cracked tooth syndrome refers to an incomplete fracture of a vital posterior tooth, with the fracture involving dentine and occasionally the pulp. The symptoms of the condition include pain on biting, or occasionally pain following chewing or clenching. The affected tooth is sometimes difficult to identify. Typically, the tooth will respond positively to vitality testing and will appear normal radiographically. Identification is, however, greatly aided by having the patient load individual teeth and, if required, separate cusps using a cotton wool roll or a Tooth Slooth fracture detector (Fig 10-11).

Cracked tooth syndrome presents mainly in patients between 30 and 50 years of age. It is classically associated with a heavily restored dentition (Fig 10-12). Men and women are equally affected. Mandibular second molars, followed by mandibular first molars and maxillary premolars, are the most

122

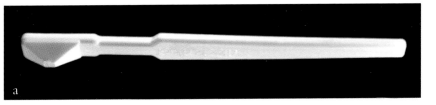

Fig 10-11 The Tooth Slooth. (a) The cup-shaped end of the instrument is designed to be placed over individual cusps of a tooth suspected of cracked tooth syndrome. (b) The patient is instructed to bite on the flat surface. Pain/discomfort is usually indicative of the presence of a cracked cusp. (b is Courtesy of the *Journal of the Canadian Dental Association*.)

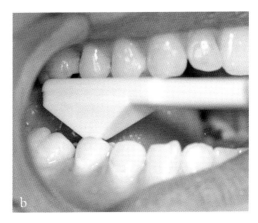

commonly affected teeth. Two classic patterns of crack formation exist. The first occurs where the crack is centrally located, following the dentinal tubules in the direction of the pulp. The second is where the crack is more peripherally directed and this may result in cuspal fracture. The pain experienced with cracked tooth syndrome is understood when considering what happens when a load is applied to the crown of a cracked tooth. Movement at the crack interface causes separation along the line of the crack.

Fig 10-12 A heavily restored tooth that the patient complained was causing discomfort on chewing. Use of the Tooth Slooth identified the presence of a cracked cusp. (Courtesy of the *Journal of the Canadian Dental Association*.)

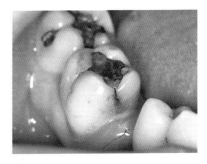

Such separation results in fluid movements in the dentinal tubules, stimulating odontoblasts in the pulp, if not stretching and rupturing odontoblastic processes, and thus stimulating pulpal nociceptors. Similarly, the pain may occur when the load is removed and the crack interface closes. Successful diagnosis of cracked tooth syndrome may be difficult. Occasionally, the crack lines may be evident if they extend along the external enamel surfaces. More often than not, the crack lines are within the body of the tooth. The orientation of the fracture lines results in symptoms in lateral loading only.

Some of the most common aetiological factors associated with cracked tooth syndrome include:
• the presence of large non-adhesive restorations
• over-preparation of cavities, in particular retentive features, leading to weakening of the remaining tooth tissue
• the placement of pins
• bulk placement of posterior composite restorations
• forced seating of a tight-fitting intracoronal casting
• unfavourable occlusal relationships
• bruxism and other parafunctional activity.

Management options for cracked tooth syndrome depend on the nature and orientation of the crack. A peripherally located crack that involves a small portion of the tooth may be removed during cavity preparation and the tooth restored using an adhesively bonded restoration. Centrally located cracks may require "stabilisation" of the tooth. Historically, stabilisation of a cracked tooth involved occlusal adjustment and the placement of an orthodontic band, followed, after an appropriate period of time, by placement of a full-coverage crown, assuming the placement of the band relieved the symptoms and the tooth remained vital.

With the developments of composite resins and associated bonding technologies, adhesively bonded composite resin restorations have tended to be used for stabilisation, with and without the use of small amounts of composite reinforcing fibres or matting being placed across the crack in the base of the cavity (Fig 10-13).

Should this "stabilisation" be successful and there are no further symptoms, there is no reason why the stabilising posterior composite cannot be regarded as the long-term management for the affected tooth. In stabilising a cracked tooth, there is always the anxiety that there has been bacterial penetration of the crack and that this eventually will lead to death of the pulp. Assuming

Fig 10-13 Use of a composite restoration to stabilise a cracked maxillary second molar. The patient presented with symptoms of cracked tooth syndrome associated with this tooth; placement of a posterior composite restoration led to resolution of the symptoms. The patient has since been symptom free for nearly two years.

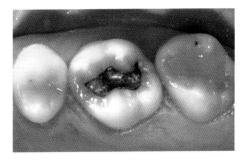

an adhesively bonded restoration is placed to stabilise the tooth and the restoration has good marginal seal, any bacterial penetration that may have occurred should not be cause for concern.

Restoring Endodontically Treated Teeth

Given the changing therapeutic paradigms in restorative dentistry, with an increased emphasis on tooth conservation, many more teeth than was previously the case are saved by means of endodontic treatment. Such treatment is of itself a highly successful means of retaining teeth; success rates in the region of 98% are reported where the treatment has been satisfactorily completed (Figs 10-14 to 10-16). In recent years, it has been recognised that a good-quality coronal seal and restoration are important to the success and survival of the endodontically treated tooth. A coronal seal is necessary to

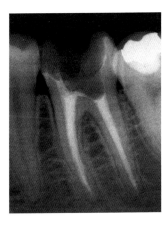

Fig 10-14 A good-quality root canal filling is critical to the success of endodontic therapy. This post-obturation radiograph was taken prior to placement of an appropriate coronal restoration.

125

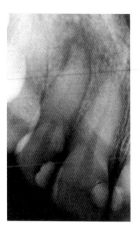

Fig 10-15 A periapical radiolucency indicative of the presence of periapical disease associated with the maxillary lateral incisor.

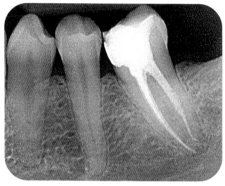

Fig 10-16 Good-quality root canal treatment can cure periapical disease. (Courtesy of Dr L Jones, Kilrush, Co. Clare, Ireland).

prevent ingress of bacteria into the root canal system and, as a consequence, the periapical tissues. Composite resin is one material that is capable of providing a good coronal seal, thereby limiting the entry of harmful bacteria. Broadly speaking, composite resins may be used in one of two ways in the restoration of endodontically treated teeth:

- the "simple" restoration of an access cavity: a four- or three-walled cavity contained within the crown of the endodontically treated tooth
- the restoration of an endodontically treated tooth that has been extensively damaged by caries, fracture or iatrogenic means.

Composite resin is indicated in the restoration of "simple" access cavities, even when made through existing direct (dental amalgam or composite resin) or indirect (metal–ceramic, metal or all-ceramic) restorations. The placement of composite restorations in such situations should not be considered any different to the placement of composite resin in cavities in vital teeth. Where gutta-percha has been used to obturate the root canal system, it should be reduced to a level just below the cementoenamel junction and then covered with a layer of resin-modified glass–ionomer cement. This helps to isolate the root filling and precludes damage to the endodontic seal during etching and subsequent bonding. Access for light curing close to the cementoenamel junction will be limited. Care is, therefore, required to ensure that the composite material is fully polymerised, in particular at the base of the cavity.

Composite resin is widely used to restore extensively damaged endodontically treated teeth, in particular those to be restored with the aid of state-of-the-art post systems and as a prelude to crowning.

The philosophy underpinning the use of posts in endodontically treated teeth has changed considerably since the mid 1980s, with a growing understanding that the purpose of a post is to help to retain and improve the biomechanical properties of a typical core for a crown. Rather than reinforcing an endodontically treated tooth, the use of a post may, through preparation and altered biomechanical behaviour, weaken the tooth. In recent times, various fibre post systems have been introduced, which are "kinder" to the affected tooth. This may be understood in light of two significant factors:
- Fibre posts have a modulus of elasticity that is closer than cast metal posts to that of dentine. Fibre posts flex with the restored tooth unit under loading, while metal posts are rigid. Given the more favourable biomechanical behaviours of the fibre posts, the risk of mechanical failure of remaining tooth tissues, let alone the interfaces of the restoration, is greatly reduced.
- Fibre posts are placed using adhesive systems rather than traditional cements and so the restored tooth unit is better able to distribute stresses under loading. Additionally, the adhesive approach affords opportunities to preserve as much remaining tooth tissue as possible.

Composite resin may be used as the sole material to restore extensively damaged endodontically treated teeth, including those that require the use of a post. The technique is especially useful when the patient cannot afford more expensive forms of restoration, such as a crown, or more generally when there is concern regarding the prognosis of the endodontically treated tooth. The clinical procedure for placing this form of restoration is little different to that used to restore extensively damaged vital teeth. There are, however, two key considerations:

- The pulp space should be restored with a glass–ionomer cement (if a post is not required) in order to help to restore the biomechanical properties of the tooth, while making the endodontic treatment retrievable. A total etch procedure would make re-entry to the pulp space, let alone the root canals, difficult.
- Endodontically treated teeth are at risk of fracture if the restored tooth is subjected to heavy loading, in particular heavy lateral loading. This may lead to the fracture of one or more cusps, and occlusal reduction with subsequent cuspal coverage is typically indicated. In the event of adopting such an approach, consideration should be given to reducing the size of the occlusal table and otherwise reducing occlusal loading through careful design of the cuspal angles and configuration.

Key Learning Points

- Composite resin is a versatile and conservative treatment option when managing worn posterior teeth.
- Adhesively bonded composite resin offers a relatively simple yet effective means of managing a posterior tooth affected by cracked tooth syndrome.
- Composite resin is the material of choice for the restoration of simple access cavities in endodontically treated teeth, and it can find application in the restoration of more extensively damaged endodontically posterior teeth.

Further Reading

Bartlett D. Using composites to restore worn teeth. J Can Dent Assoc 2006;72:301–304.

Lynch CD, McConnell RJ. The cracked tooth syndrome. J Can Dent Assoc 2002;68:470–475.

Lynch CD, Burke FM, Ní Riordan R, Hannigan A. The influence of coronal restoration type on the survival of endodontically treated teeth. Eur J Prosthodont Restor Dent 2004;12:171–176.

Ray HA, Trope M. Periapical status of endodontically treated teeth in relation to the technical quality of the root filling and coronal restoration. Int Endodont J 1995;28:12–18.

Chapter 11

When Things Go Wrong: Trouble-shooting Posterior Composites

Aim

This aim of this chapter is to consider some of the common post-treatment problems that can occur with posterior composites, and to advise on the management and prevention of such difficulties.

Outcome

Having read this chapter, the reader will be familiar with the presentation and management of post-treatment problems associated with posterior composites, including sensitivity, restoration fracture, discoloration, loss of marginal integrity, food packing and loss of pulp vitality.

Introduction

The placement of posterior composite restorations is demanding. Notwithstanding the technical challenges of achieving an optimal clinical outcome, there are risks of post-operative complications.

In general, most post-operative problems with posterior composites relate to inappropriate handling of the material or to the use of operative techniques that are less than ideal. This is often coupled with a lack of understanding of the physical properties and limitations of the materials used. Examples of operator-related factors include:
- inappropriate management of operatively exposed dentine
- bulk- placement and curing of composite materials with a lack of understanding of the need for incremental curing
- treatment of dentine in a similar manner to enamel, with no provision for the unique structure and composition of dentine, let alone the status of the dentine in individual cases.

When the Worst Happens: What Can Go Wrong

Some common post-treatment problems that can occur in relation to posterior composites include:

- persistent post-treatment sensitivity
- restoration fracture, either bulk or marginal fracture
- loss of retention
- discoloration
- loss of marginal integrity
- food packing associated with proximal composite restorations
- pulp death.

Post-treatment Sensitivity

Post-treatment sensitivity is perhaps one of the most frustrating and difficult problems that occur in relation to posterior composite restorations. The possible causes of the sensitivity are multifactorial, and may include:

- leakage
- stressing or flexure of cusps and cavity walls
- enamel cracking and development of cracked tooth syndrome
- over-etching of dentine
- over-drying of dentine
- inadvertent etching of exposed cervical areas
- retention of etchant below a poorly placed or inappropriate, non-adhesive base
- insufficient or under-powered light curing
- inappropriate occlusal contacts.

As will be noted from this list, the aetiology of post-treatment sensitivity relates mainly to procedural errors, be it failure to manage operatively exposed dentine appropriately, an inappropriate operative technique or a failure to diagnose an existing problem, such as cracked tooth syndrome. This list serves as a reminder of the central tenets of posterior composite restoration placement outlined earlier in this book, notably the advice that composite is not tooth-coloured amalgam and should not be handled as such, and that dentine and enamel are very dissimilar tissues and respond differently to the materials and techniques to which they are exposed.

Playing the blame game

The successful management of post-treatment sensitivity depends in the first instance on identifying the likely cause of the problem. A careful history should be recorded, with a special emphasis on the length of time that the restoration has been in place, and the characteristics of the symptoms experienced, such as its nature, severity and duration. Pain unrelated to the restoration, including pulpal inflammation in adjacent teeth or pain of periodontal or non-odontogenic origin, should be excluded. Attention should then focus on the clinical examination, which should include an assessment of the adjacent teeth for the presence of caries or defective restorations, as well as an examination of the occlusal relationships to check for any interferences.

Identifying the likely cause of post-treatment sensitivity can sometimes be difficult, in particular if it is caused by "flexed" or "stressed" cusps. On occasion, the diagnosis may be aided by applying a layer of bonding resin, or so-called "desensitising resin", to the margins of the restoration giving rise to the problem. If this reduces or stops the symptoms, then the cause of the problem is most likely to be leakage. If the relief from the symptoms is complete, then no further treatment may be indicated; if the problem recurs, then it is usually necessary to replace the restoration with meticulous care being given to the placement technique, mindful that there had been some failure in the initial attempt to restore the tooth.

Other diagnostic tests of use in identifying the cause of post-treatment sensitivity include the use of articulating paper to investigate the presence of any inappropriate occlusal or excursive contacts, the use of a Tooth Slooth or other so-called "bite-tests" to identify stressed or cracked cusps, transillumination to identify cracks and radiographs to identify major deficiencies and possibly voids in the restoration, depending on the radio-opacity of the material. Caution is advised when reading radiographs of teeth restored with posterior composites, as a thick layer of a radiolucent dentine-bonding agent or a radiolucent base may be confused with poor adaptation or secondary caries.

In the event of post-treatment sensitivity persisting more than a few days and being difficult to diagnose, arrangements should be made to remove the restoration to allow detailed inspection of the remaining tooth structure with the aid of illumination and magnification. This permits investigation for the presence of, in particular, crack lines, residual caries or a pulpal exposure that escaped radiographic diagnosis. Given that the tooth will be best protected by a bonded restoration, a new composite restoration should be placed, but with great care being taken throughout the operative procedure, including effective dentine management, incremental placing and curing, the avoidance of polymerisation stresses and atraumatic finishing. The patient should then be discharged but with instructions to return in the event of any recurrence of the symptoms.

131

Posterior composites that give rise to intermittent post-operative sensitivity are better replaced than modified in some way. If intermittent sensitivity eventually fades away, this is usually indicative of deterioration in the status of the pulp.

Restoration Fracture
Possible reasons for the fracture of a posterior composite restoration include:
- an inappropriate occlusal contact left in the restoration
- failure to identify pre-existing parafunctional loading
- exceptional, unforeseen loading on biting down on a hard item of food or foreign body
- an adverse change in loading subsequent to a change in the function of adjacent or opposing teeth
- incomplete polymerisation of the restoration at the time of placement, caused by either the placement of excessively thick increments or the use of a poor light curing technique
- the presence of a large void in the body of the restoration
- the use of a thick cement base, which reduces the fracture resistance of the restoration.

Appropriate management of a fractured restoration again depends on identifying the reason for the failure. The fracture can be simply treated by repairing the existing restoration (Chapter 9), but performing a repair without having identified and managed the underlying problem typically invites recurrence of the failure.

Loss of Retention
Loss of retention can be an embarrassing outcome, in particular if the treatment was offered to the patient on the grounds that it is adhesive in nature. Again, successful management of this complication is dependent on identifying the cause. Possible reasons for loss of retention of a posterior composite include:
- failure to etch enamel and dentine appropriately
- failure to apply the bonding agent appropriately; the manufacturer's directions for use must be followed
- contamination of either the etched or "bonded" tooth surfaces
- inadequate polymerisation of the composite material
- incorporation of an inappropriate occlusal or excursive contact in the completed restoration
- fracture of the tooth, typically a cusp followed by loss of the restoration
- failure to identify a parafunctional habit.

Treatment for this difficulty is to place a new restoration, with meticulous attention to detail. The design of the cavity may need to be modified to enhance the "bonding form" of the preparation.

Discoloration

Discoloration, be it of the margins of the restoration or "in bulk", can be an undesired complication in the provision of tooth-coloured restorations. Some possible causes include:

- failure to polish the surfaces of the completed restoration adequately
- dietary or "habitual" causes, including cigarette smoking or excessive dietary intake of coffee, tea or red wine
- damage of the restoration or its margins during finishing, for example by the use of stones that tend to fracture the margins of the restoration, or as a consequence of excessive heat generation during the use of rotary instrumentation.

Discoloration of the surface or margins of a posterior composite restoration is not necessarily an indication to replace the restoration, especially if the restoration is relatively new and otherwise clinically satisfactory. If, however, the patient is concerned with the appearance of the stained restoration, it is acceptable to perform a refurbishment procedure, whereby the superficial stained layer is removed, and a fresh layer of composite material is added.

Loss of Marginal Integrity

Loss of marginal integrity is an occasional problem found in association with posterior composites. It may occur in association with post-treatment sensitivity. The reasons for loss of marginal integrity may include:

- inappropriate placement technique, where the composite material is inadequately sculpted to the cavity cavosurface margins
- inappropriate curing technique associated with excessive polymerisation; contraction results in the creation of a marginal gap or creates stresses within the marginal composite that subsequently fractures under occlusal loading
- bevelling of the occlusal cavosurface margins, resulting in thin extensions of composite resin being incorporated into the completed restoration; under repeated occlusal loading, these extensions, as well as some neighbouring composite from the bulk of the completed restoration, may fracture away
- damage of the restoration margins during finishing
- the margin of the restoration being left directly under an occlusal contact.

If loss of marginal integrity occurs in association with post-treatment sensitivity, then a suitable management strategy, such as the application of a "de-sensitising" bonding agent or localised refurbishment, should be instituted. Disruption of marginal integrity is, of itself, not an indication to replace a posterior composite. Some form of operative intervention is typically indicated, however, as marginal integrity will tend to deteriorate further if left unattended.

Food Packing

Food packing in association with a proximal composite restoration reflects a failure to adequately restore the proximal contour or an effective proximal contact point, or the creation of a proximal overhang. A dental explorer can be used to detect the presence of proximal overhangs, and the adequacy of the proximal contact point can be assessed using dental floss. The presence of proximal overhangs may also be detected using bitewing radiography, assuming the composite material is sufficiently radio-opaque. Successful management of food packing depends on correctly identifying its cause. Should a proximal overhang be present, then this can often be removed using appropriate instrumentation, though it is generally more appropriate to replace the proximal portion of the restoration if the overhang is substantial or deeply placed. For an open or inadequate proximal contact, the proximal portion of the restoration may be replaced (Chapter 7); the "new" proximal area should be restored using a precontoured, sectional metal matrix and flexible/wooden wedge. As described in Chapter 7, the composite material should be adapted and sculpted incrementally to the internal features of the cavity and matrix, and the missing proximal wall restored prior to placing the body of the restoration.

Loss of Pulpal Vitality

Loss of pulpal vitality can occur with any form of restorative material. Teeth appropriately restored with composite resin are not at a higher risk of pulp death. Composite resin is not of itself toxic to pulpal cells; pulpal necrosis is a consequence of bacterial invasion, be it from a failure to remove all the caries during the placement of the initial restoration, the subsequent ingress of bacteria (leakage) or the formation of a secondary caries. However, "at risk" teeth include those with restorations that are close to the pulp and those that were restored using a direct or indirect pulp-capping technique.

In the event of the death of the pulp, the presence of a large composite resin restoration does not limit the ability to perform endodontic treatment.

Key Learning Points

- Post-treatment problems occasionally occur in association with posterior composites.
- Many post-treatment problems can be prevented by careful and appropriate handling of the composite material, bonding systems and underlying tooth structure.
- When managing post-treatment problems, it is critical that the cause of the problem, for example an inappropriate excursive occlusal contact, is identified to avoid incorporating the same error in the replaced/refurbished restoration.
- If problems persist, the restoration should be replaced.

Chapter 12

Don't Always Believe What You Read in Books: A Critique of Posterior Composites

Aim

The aim of this chapter is to revisit some of the concepts discussed in this book, with an emphasis on the evidence base for some of the more contentious aspects of posterior composite resin restorations. The concepts are dealt with in the style of questions (Q) and answers (A).

Outcome

Having read this chapter, the reader will be familiar with current best evidence and the practice guidelines pertaining to the placement of posterior composite resin restorations.

Concepts and Critical Issues

Q: *Are composite resins the material of choice for the restoration of conservative cavities prepared in accordance with the principles of minimally interventive dentistry?*
A: Yes. Apart from requiring more extensive cavity preparation, dental amalgam is difficult to manipulate and, importantly, condense in conservative, let alone ultraconservative, cavities. In contrast, in addition to their good bonding and sealing capabilities, composite resins can achieve full restoration when handled appropriately and adapt well to minimally interventive cavity forms. Composite resins should be viewed as the material of choice for, in particular, initial minimally interventive restorations in posterior teeth.

Q: *Do posterior composite restorations survive for as long as restorations of dental amalgam?*
A: Yes. In an increasing range of situations, the development of sophisticated composite resin materials and adhesive technologies, in association with an improved understanding of the appropriate application and handling of these materials, means that well-placed posterior composite restorations can survive for at least as long as equivalent restorations using dental amalgam. Furthermore, composite resin restorations offer much more than dental amalgam in terms of restoring the biomechanical features of the tooth and

they can be repaired and refurbished in clinical service, limiting the need for repeated restoration replacement as part of routine dental care.

Q: *Do I need to use a rubber dam when placing posterior composites?*
A: No, not always. Current evidence suggests that the quality of isolation achieved is more important that the clinical technique selected. It has been demonstrated that posterior composite restorations placed in situations in which adequate isolation was achieved with, for example, cotton wool rolls and high-volume aspiration have comparable longevity to posterior composites placed with the use of rubber dam. Notwithstanding such findings, a well-placed rubber dam retracts and protects soft tissues, facilitates washing and drying of the preparation and eliminates salivary aerosol in the working environment. A badly placed rubber dam can be more hindrance than help in the placement of posterior composites.

Q: *Can I use the same cavity design for posterior composites and dental amalgam?*
A: No. Composite resins should not be regarded as a substitute or replacement for dental amalgam. They require different operative procedures including different cavity design and preparation. When placing composite resin, it is often sufficient to remove the soft, infected carious dentine, and to finish the margins of the preparation prior to proceeding to restoration placement. In contrast, it is necessary to excavate back to hard, albeit stained, dentine when using dental amalgam and to perform various cavity modifications, often further compromising the strength of the tooth.

Q: *Should I bevel occlusal cavity margins prior to placing a posterior composite?*
A: No. The occlusal cavosurface cavity margins should not be finished with a long, low bevel as is used in anterior restorations. If a long, low bevel were placed, it would lead to the formation of thin extensions of composite resin on the load-bearing occlusal surface of the restored tooth. Such thin extensions are liable to fracture under direct loading, compromising the marginal integrity of the restoration. Bevelled margins will also create difficulties when the restoration needs to be refurbished, repaired or replaced; it may be difficult to identify the extent of the existing restoration, which may lead to the unnecessary removal of intact tooth tissue. Cavity preparation appropriate for posterior composites will leave margins with an intra–enamel bevel sufficient to enhance bonding and, in turn, achieve a favourable marginal seal.

Q: *Is it safe to etch dentine?*
A: Yes, provided care is taken to use a proprietary etchant strictly in accordance with the manufacturer's directions. Dentine, unlike enamel, is

a vital tissue. While etching of dentine removes the smear layer and exposes the limiting layer of collagen fibres to contribute to hybrid layer formation, over-etching dentine can cause post-treatment sensitivity and compromise bonding. When etchant is used according to the manufacturer's directions, the pulpal reaction to etching is limited and transitory, even when the remaining dentinal thickness is substantially reduced.

Q: *When managing moderately deep and deep cavities in posterior teeth, should I place a base prior to restoring the tooth with a composite resin?*
A: This, to many, is a contentious issue. While there is no clinical evidence to suggest superior outcomes are achieved when, for example, a resin-modified glass–ionomer cement base has been placed, many clinicians continue this practice, possibly as a form of defensive dentistry. Such an approach to the management of exposed dentine flies in the face of the evidence, which indicates that newer dentine bonding agents have the ability to seal exposed dentinal tubules and cavity margins reliably while optimising the performance of the completed composite restoration. The use of a cement base limits the area available for adhesive bonding and reduces the thickness of the overlying restoration. This reduced thickness will compromise the fracture resistance of the completed restoration, possibly increasing the risk of bulk fracture in clinical service.

Q: *Should I use a pin to retain a large posterior composite restoration?*
A: Absolutely not. The use of dentine pins should be avoided wherever possible. Current best-available research has consistently demonstrated that the use of dentine pins is associated with the localised concentration of stresses within the restored tooth, with the risk of iatrogenic damage to the pulp or periodontal ligament. Dentine pins are now an outmoded and outdated aid to retention, particularly with the availability of predictable and highly successful dentine bonding systems.

Q: *What factors should I consider when selecting a composite material for placement in a posterior cavity?*
A: Whatever resin material is selected, its filler:resin ratio by volume should exceed 60%. These materials, typically hybrids with a mixture of fillers of different sizes, have sufficient compressive strength and wear resistance to function adequately in most posterior situations. Other factors include the polymerisation contraction of the selected material. A material that features limited contraction will be advantageous, though polymerisation contraction can largely be overcome with a careful placement technique. The use of flowable resins is not recommended, as these materials tend to be associated

with relatively high polymerisation contraction and poor marginal integrity. Where aesthetic demands permit, it is advantageous to select a composite material of a slightly lighter shade to the tooth being restored. This will help to limit iatrogenic damage to adjacent enamel during finishing and, in time, facilitate refurbishment, repair or replacement by allowing differentiation between the restoration and the remaining tooth tissues.

Q: *What is the best light-curing unit to use when placing posterior composites?*
A: It is critical to the success of posterior composites to use a light-curing unit capable of delivering light of the appropriate quantity and intensity for the required time in order to polymerise the material. Quartz halogen–tungsten and light-emitting diode (LED) units are suitable for this purpose, while plasma arc lights are of limited value. The LED units have the advantage of being more energy efficient, portable and increasingly more powerful than the quartz halogen–tungsten units. It is anticipated that the use of LED units will become widespread in coming years.

Q: *What is the best placement technique for posterior composite restorations?*
A: Selection of an appropriate placement technique is critical to the success of a completed posterior composite restoration. It is crucial to realise that composite resin is not tooth–coloured dental amalgam, and so must not be handled using amalgam techniques. Composite resin must not be bulk placed or bulk cured in a cavity; it also should not be condensed or otherwise manipulated like dental amalgam in a cavity. Composite resin should be directly injected into the cavity and sculpted as little as possible, with the restoration being built up in successive increments of not greater than 2 mm thickness. Increments should not link opposing cusps or cavity walls. They should be placed in oblique layers, thereby limiting the build up of contraction stresses in the restored tooth unit. Superior clinical outcomes have been observed when the composite resin material is delivered into the cavity directly from compules, rather than being carried into the cavity with instruments. Preheating techniques for compules have been considered advantageous in terms of facilitating the placement of composites. Placing instruments should have highly polished damage-free functional surfaces. Under no circumstances should the tips of placement instruments be dipped in alcohol, resin, water or any other medium to reduce sticking to composites.

Q: *Why is depth of cure important?*
A: Failure to take account of the depth of cure of the selected material will result in inadequate polymerisation in the deepest regions of the restoration.

140

This will be difficult to detect clinically, as the superficial, accessible layers of the material will, as a consequence of being closer to the light-curing tip, be adequately polymerised. Inadequate polymerisation of the deepest regions of a restoration may give rise to post-treatment sensitivity, with longer-term problems such as bulk discoloration, restoration fracture and recurrent caries. Generally, the irradiation of an increment of composite resin of 2 mm thickness for 30 seconds will ensure adequate polymerisation. Reduced depth of cure is associated with darker shades of composite resin, increased distance between the tip of the light-curing guide and the composite material, a reduced power output of the light-curing unit and shorter curing times. The thickness of the increments placed should be adjusted to take account of these factors.

Q: *What is the best matrix and wedge system for placing proximal composite restorations?*
A: A sectional, or in some situations a circumferential metal matrix, adapted with a flexible/wooden wedge gives the most favourable outcome. However, careful consideration needs to be given to the placement technique in order to restore the proximal contact area and to avoid the formation of proximal overhangs. A useful technique is first to create the missing proximal wall and then to restore the remainder of the proximal region as if it were an "occlusal"/four-walled cavity. The completed restoration should be additionally cured buccally and lingually following removal of the matrix. Transparent matrix bands and light-transmitting wedges are to be avoided because of their thick and relatively stiff nature. Current evidence suggests that sectional metal matrices may achieve superior clinical results compared with circumferential metal matrices.

Q: *What factors do I need to remember when finishing posterior composite restorations?*
A: The techniques selected for finishing posterior composite restorations can have a significant effect on the subsequent performance of the restored tooth unit. The use of a water coolant is recommended as this reduces the amount of heat generated in the completed restoration while rinsing away debris and permitting better visual access to the operation site. The use of magnification is also recommended as a means of further reducing the risk of iatrogenic damage to the surrounding enamel.

Q: *Is it acceptable to repair damaged or fractured posterior composite restorations with "fresh" composite resin?*
A: Yes, repair of existing posterior composite restorations is considered preferable to restoration replacement in many situations. However, each case

141

needs to be carefully assessed. A repair is contraindicated in the presence of extensive secondary caries, a history of failure of previous repairs and failure by the patient to give informed consent for the procedure.

Q: *Is the use of composite resins in the restoration of posterior teeth likely to increase?*
A: Yes, the future of operative dentistry lies in prevention, minimally invasive techniques and the use of tooth-coloured restorative systems, including the use of composite resin in the restoration of posterior teeth. The rate of increase in the use of composite resins in the restoration of posterior teeth is accelerating, with a concurrent reduction in the use of traditional materials, notably dental amalgam. The trend towards the increasing use of composite resins for the restoration of posterior teeth is global.

Index

Quintessentials for General Dental Practitioners Series

in 11 volumes

Editor-in-Chief: Professor Nairn H F Wilson

The Quintessentials for General Dental Practitioners Series covers basic principles and key issues in all aspects of modern dental medicine. Each book can be read as a stand-alone volume or in conjunction with other books in the series.

	Publication date, approximately
Clinical Practice, Editor: Nairn Wilson	
Culturally Sensitive Oral Healthcare	available
Dental Erosion	available
Special Care Dentistry	available
Evidence-based Dentistry	available
Infection Control for the Dental Team	Summer 2008
Oral Surgery and Oral Medicine, Editor: John G Meechan	
Practical Dental Local Anaesthesia	available
Practical Oral Medicine	available
Practical Conscious Sedation	available
Minor Oral Surgery in Dental Practice	available
Imaging, Editor: Keith Horner	
Interpreting Dental Radiographs	available
Panoramic Radiology	available
21st Century Dental Imaging	available
Periodontology, Editor: Iain L C Chapple	
Understanding Periodontal Diseases: Assessment and Diagnostic Procedures in Practice	available
Decision-Making for the Periodontal Team	available
Successful Periodontal Therapy – A Non-Surgical Approach	available
Periodontal Management of Children, Adolescents and Young Adults	available
Periodontal Medicine: A Window on the Body	available
Contemporary Periodontal Surgery – An Illustrated Guide to the Art Behind the Science	available

Endodontics, Editor: John M Whitworth

    Rational Root Canal Treatment in Practice   available
    Managing Endodontic Failure in Practice   available
    Adhesive Restoration of Endodontically Treated Teeth   available

Prosthodontics, Editor: P Finbarr Allen

    Teeth for Life for Older Adults   available
    Complete Dentures – from Planning to Problem Solving   available
    Removable Partial Dentures   available
    Fixed Prosthodontics in Dental Practice   available
    Applied Occlusion   available
    Orofacial Pain: A Guide for General Practitioners   available

Operative Dentistry, Editor: Paul A Brunton

    Decision-Making in Operative Dentistry   available
    Aesthetic Dentistry   available
    Communicating in Dental Practice   available
    Indirect Restorations   available
    Dental Bleaching   available
    Dental Materials in Operative Dentistry   available
    Successful Posterior Composites   available

Paediatric Dentistry/Orthodontics, Editor: Marie Therese Hosey

    Child Taming: How to Manage Children in Dental Practice   available
    Paediatric Cariology   available
    Treatment Planning for the Developing Dentition   available
    Managing Dental Trauma in Practice   available

General Dentistry and Practice Management, Editor: Raj Rattan

    The Business of Dentistry   available
    Risk Management in General Dental Practice   available
    Quality Matters: From Clinical Care to Customer Service   available

Dental Team, Editor: Mabel Slater

    Team Players in Dentistry   Summer 2008

Implantology, Editor: Lloyd J Searson

    Implantology in General Dental Practice   available

Quintessence Publishing Co. Ltd., London